DERMATOLOGY

MANAGEMENT OF COMMON DISEASES IN FAMILY PRACTICE

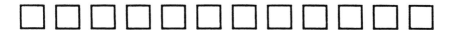

Series Editors: J. Fry and M. Lancaster-Smith

DERMATOLOGY

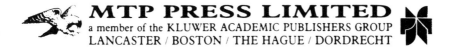

L. Fry, BSc, MD, FRCP

Consultant Dermatologist,
St. Mary's Hospital, London

and

M. N. P. Cornell, MRCP, DCH, DRCOG

General Practitioner, Bayswater

MTP PRESS LIMITED
a member of the KLUWER ACADEMIC PUBLISHERS GROUP
LANCASTER / BOSTON / THE HAGUE / DORDRECHT

Published in the UK and Europe by
MTP Press Limited
Falcon House
Lancaster, England

British Library Cataloguing in Publication Data

Fry, L.
  Dermatology — (Management of common diseases in family practice)
  1. Skin — Diseases
  I. Title   II. Cornell, M. N. P.   III. Title
  616.5   RL71

  ISBN 0-85200-890-2
  ISBN 0-85200-794-9 Set

Typeset by UPS Blackburn, 76–80 Northgate, Blackburn, Lancashire and
Printed and Bound in Great Britain by Butler & Tanner Ltd, Frome and London.

Contents

□ □ □ □ □ □ □ □ □ □ □

Colour figures may be found between pages 104 and 105.

Series Editors' Foreword

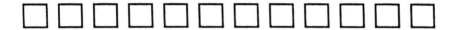

Effective management logically follows accurate diagnosis. Such logic often is difficult to apply in practice. Absolute diagnostic accuracy may not be possible, particularly in the field of primary care, when management has to be on analysis of symptoms and on knowledge of the individual patient and family.

This series follows that on *Problems in Practice* which was concerned more with diagnosis in the widest sense and this series deals more definitively with general care and specific treatment of symptoms and diseases.

Good management must include knowledge of the nature, course and outcome of the conditions, as well as prominent clinical features and assessment and investigations, but the emphasis is on what to do best for the patient.

Family medical practitioners have particular difficulties and advantages in their work. Because they often work in professional isolation in the community and deal with relatively small numbers of near-normal patients their experience with the more serious and more rare conditions is restricted. They find it difficult to remain up-to-date with medical advances and even more difficult to decide on the suitability and application of new and relatively untried methods compared with those that are 'old' and well proven.

Their advantages are that because of long-term continuous care for their patients they have come to know them and their families well and are able to become familiar with the more common and less serious diseases of their communities.

This series aims to correct these disadvantages by providing practical information and advice on the less common, potentially serious conditions, but at the same time to take note of the special features of general medical practice.

To achieve these objectives, the *titles* are intentionally those of accepted body systems and population groups.

The *co-authors* are a specialist and a family practitioner so that each can supplement and complement the other.

The *experience bases* are those of the district general hospital and family practice. It is here that the day-to-day problems arise.

The *advice and presentation* are practical and have come from many years of conjoint experience of family and hospital practice.

The *series* is intended for family practitioners – the young and the less than young. All should benefit and profit from comparing the views of the authors with their own. Many will coincide, some will be accepted as new, useful and worthy of application and others may not be acceptable, but nevertheless will stimulate thought and enquiry.

Since medical care in the community and in hospitals involves teamwork, this series also should be of relevance to nurses and others involved in personal and family care.

JOHN FRY
M. LANCASTER-SMITH

1

VIRAL INFECTIONS

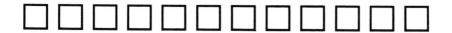

HERPES SIMPLEX

Introduction

This is a common viral disease occurring throughout the world, with up to 60% of various population groups being infected or remaining carriers.

Herpes simplex is a DNA-containing virus, Type 1 causing orofacial lesions and Type 2 causing genital lesions, with either type causing lesions elsewhere in the body; primary lesions may also involve the eyes, upper respiratory tract and central nervous system (c.n.s.), and in debilitated patients may become disseminated.

After a person has recoverd from a skin infection, the virus may lie dormant in the cells of the sensory nerves, where it may be activated by such trigger factors as high fever, exposure to sunlight and wind, stress, general debility and respiratory infection.

Transmission of the disease is essentially by direct contact and possibly by droplet. The incubation period is usually 4 – 5 days, but may be up to 3 weeks.

Infection in the first 6 months of life is rare, due to passive transfer of maternal immunity. From 6 months to 5 years, the primary infection is usually acute and affects gums, buccal mucosa and tongue. From age 5 to age 14 the primary infection is usually on the skin around the lips and eyes, and occasionally on the fingers (herpetic whitlow). Primary genital infection is most likely to present between the ages of 14 and 29, more commonly in women. Recurrent or secondary herpes simplex can occur in any of these sites.

Clinical features

The lesions are characterized by an area of erythema with superimposed vesicles which later become pustules and then crusted. There may be associated lymphadenopathy. Primary lesions are often acute and painful, although primary genital lesions may be subclinical and unnoticed. Recurrent or secondary herpes simplex infection in any site is usually heralded by a tingling sensation in the affected area.

Complications include secondary infection, localised lymphoedema, trigeminal neuralgia, keratoconjunctivitis, corneal ulcers and erythema multiforme. Occasionally, as in the severely debilitated or immunologically compromised, the infection may become generalized and involve the c.n.s. Severe spreading infection may occur in sufferers of atopic eczema, where the condition is known as Kaposi's varicelliform eruption.

Healing of primary lesions takes up to 3 weeks, but secondary lesions tend to clear in about 7–10 days.

Problems

Diagnosis may cause difficulty.

Primary herpetic gingivostomatitis should be differentiated from oral lesions of Stevens–Johnson syndrome, streptococcal infections, Coxsackie infection, Behçet's syndrome, and even thrush.

Impetigo may be mistaken for secondary infected herpes simplex, but lesions are usually more superficial. A small area of vesiculating contact eczema may cause confusion. Herpes zoster lesions are distinguished by dermatomal grouping. Occasionally scabies, monilia and fixed drug eruptions can cause confusion in diagnosis.

The more indurated syphilitic ulcer or chancre must be differentiated from the genital herpetic ulcer. Indeed, all cases of genital herpes should be investigated for other possible concurrent genitourinary disease. In addition it has been postulated that recurrent cervical herpes may be a precursor of carcinoma of the cervix; vigilant cervical screening should therefore be carried out in these cases.

Contrary to popular belief, many people who suffer an attack of genital herpes do not have recurrences, but on the other hand recurrent genital herpes may be very distressing, with frequent painful attacks associated with dysuria. Why some individuals are more susceptible than others to such attacks is not yet understood. Necessary abstinence from sexual intercourse during attacks and anxiety about overall risk of transmission may lead to psychological problems and associated stigma.

Assessment and investigation

Diagnosis is usually made on history and clinical features, but tissue culture of fluid from a vesicle can confirm the diagnosis within 4 days. Serum antibodies start rising 7 days after infection, peak in 2–3 weeks and then gradually fall to a plateau, subsequent attacks causing slight increase in antibody levels.

Management

Mild recurrent attacks may not require treatment, though various barrier preparations such as 1% aqueous zinc sulphate may be helpful. Antiseptic and antibiotic applications may be useful in cases of secondary infection.

Acyclovir (Zovirax) is a relatively new drug available in topical, oral and intravenous form. It appears to reduce the period of infectivity during which virus shedding occurs, reducing duration of symptoms and improving healing rate, but unfortunately it does not stop recurrences. Acyclovir is only effective if begun within 24 hours of the commencement of the symptoms. The oral dose is 200 mg 5 times a day for 5 days, and topically it is used as a 5% ointment applied 4 times a day. The routine use of acyclovir for uncomplicated attacks is not recommended.

Treatment of recurrent genital herpes is difficult and at present limited. General support, thorough explanation and discussion, often in collaboration with a specialist in genitourinary medicine, is required.

At present the only effective approach to the serious complication of active herpes infection in pregnancy is to deliver the baby by caesarean section.

HERPES ZOSTER

Introduction

This is a common disease caused by the varicella zoster virus, which has usually been lying dormant in a sensory root ganglion following chickenpox, being activated when immunity is impaired – although at times there seems to be no obvious reason for reactivation. The virus travels down the sensory nerve from the ganglion, causing pain to precede the eruption in the distribution of the nerve (Figure 1)*. Contact with cases of herpes zoster may cause chickenpox if the subject has not previously had the infection.

Clinical features

The dermatomal rash, following 2–3 days of pain, consists of erythematous and oedematous areas with superimposed grouped papules which become blisters, and in severe cases, haemorrhagic

* Colour figures may be found between pages 104 and 105.

or necrotic. The lesions form scabs after 7–10 days, and then gradually heal. There may be associated lymphadenopathy and constitutional upset. The common dermatome affected is thoracic.

With involvement of the ophthalmic division of trigeminal nerve, there is a 50% chance of complications affecting the eye, such as keratitis, iridocyclitis and ulcers of cornea and conjunctiva.

Involvement of ciliary ganglion may give rise to the Argyll–Robertson pupil. Involvement of the maxillary division of trigeminal nerve causes lesions on cheek and uvular and tonsillar areas. Involvement of the mandibular division will likewise produce lesions on anterior tongue, floor of mouth and buccal mucosa, as well as on skin over the neck and jaw. Geniculate ganglion involvement may cause painful lesions on the pinna and in the external auditory canal, and on the anterior two thirds of tongue. Occasionally this is part of the Ramsay Hunt syndrome with associated facial palsy.

The virus rarely affects the anterior horn cells of the corresponding sensory ganglion causing paresis. Herpes zoster myelitis and encephalitis are also rare, as is spreading generalized infection associated with abnormal immune status such as in reticuloses.

The most common complications of herpes zoster are *secondary infection and post-herpetic neuralgia,* the latter being particularly common in the elderly, when it may persist for months or even years.

Problems

Occasionally pain is severe and constitutional disturbance is very debilitating and patients require extra care.

Differential diagnosis is usually not a problem, but occasionally unilateral patches of herpes simplex, contact eczema or erysipelas cause confusion.

Other difficulties involve treatment of ophthalmic zoster, and post-herpetic neuralgia, debility and depression.

Assessment and investigation

Diagnosis is usually made on clinical grounds, but fluid from an early blister can be taken for tissue culture if necessary. Serum antibody titres are not very helpful because of previous chickenpox infection.

Management

Symptomatic treatment is required in most cases, and relatively few cases need more than moderate analgesia and rest. If applied early enough, 5% idoxuridine in dimethyl sulphoxide may decrease the severity of the attack. The lotion is applied at 4-hourly intervals for 2 days, as soon as the blisters appear. Oral acyclovir 200 mg 5 times a day for 5 days has been claimed to shorten the attack if begun in the first 24 hours of the skin lesions appearing. Topical antiseptics and antibiotics should be used if secondary infection occurs.

Eye involvement should be dealt with by the ophthalmologist. Generalized and systemic involvement may be helped by acyclovir.

Post-herpetic neuralgia is very difficult to treat. Therapies range from simple ethyl chloride sprays to surgical procedures to sever pain fibres in the spinal cord and destruction of the trigeminal ganglion with alcohol injection. Strong analgesics, to which addiction or dependency may develop, are best avoided.

HAND, FOOT AND MOUTH DISEASE

Introduction

This is a sporadic or epidemic viral disease occurring throughout the world and affecting mostly children under the age of 10. Various types of Coxsackie virus are responsible.

Clinical features

After 3–5 days incubation there is fever and soreness in the mouth, followed by a vesicular eruption on tongue, gums, buccal mucosa, palms, soles and occasionally fingers. The vesicles are small, with surrounding erythema; they rupture to cause shallow ulcers which resolve in 3–4 days without scarring. In atopic subjects the eruption may be more severe and resemble Kaposi's varicelliform eruption.

Problems

Differential diagnosis may be difficult. Herpangina is also due to Coxsackie virus, but illness is more severe with abdominal pains and vomiting; the lesions are further back in the mouth on fauces, tonsils and pharynx, and there is no skin involvement.

Herpes simplex as primary infection may present with oral ulceration, but lesions are usually further forward in the mouth and involving perioral skin. Aphthous ulcers typically have a yellow base and are not associated with constitutional upset or lesions on the skin. A mild case of Stevens–Johnson syndrome, and early secondary syphilis rash, may also cause confusion.

Assessment and investigation

Diagnosis can usually be made on clinical grounds, but virus can be isolated from the faeces. Blood count and film show lymphocytosis and monocytosis with atypical cells in the peripheral blood. Serum may show increasing titre of neutralizing antibodies.

Management

This is entirely symptomatic once a definite diagnosis has been made, and the condition is self-limiting and rarely lasts more than 1 week.

MOLLUSCUM CONTAGIOSUM

Introduction

This is a common condition caused by a pox virus resulting in papular lesions mostly on trunk, hands and anogenital areas. Mucous membranes may be affected, especially in the oral cavity. The condition is more prevalent in childhood. In adults the genital area is more typically involved. Transmission is by direct contact.

Clinical features

Following inoculation there is incubation lasting from 2 to several weeks, followed by solitary or multiple lesions, consisting of dome-shaped papules with central umbilication which may contain a caseous plug. The papule is firm and pearl coloured (Figure 2); it enlarges to 5–10 mm, and then softens. New crops of lesions may occur as a result of auto-inoculation. The disease is self-limiting with spontaneous remission usually within a year, but in some individuals lesions persist for a number of years.

Problems

The important differential diagnosis is from the nodulocystic forms of basal cell carcinoma which typically have an uneven surface with telangectasia, and no umbilication, the tumour being more usually solitary. Pyogenic granuloma is a vascular tumour that is reddish and tends to erode and bleed. Keratoacanthomata tend to be larger than molluscum contagiosa and have a central horny plug.

Assessment and investigation

Diagnosis is usually made on clinical grounds, but if there is any doubt, curettage should be followed by histology.

Management

The lesions can be removed by curettage and cautery or be pierced by a sharpened orange stick dipped in 1% phenol. They may also be treated by application of liquid nitrogen or caustics such as 5% podophyllin and 5% salicylic acid in collodion, but not near the eyes.

WARTS

Introduction

Warts are epithelial tumours caused by the papova group of viruses. Transmission is by direct or indirect contact and auto-inoculation. Warts are most common in schoolchildren.

Clinical features

The common wart is a small, rounded, elevated tumour with a horny surface. Plane warts are smaller, flesh coloured and flat. Plantar warts are deepseated, firm, hyperkeratotic lesions that may be single or multiple, or coalesce to form the mosaic wart. Condylomata acuminata are genital warts, usually flesh-coloured, pedunculated or filiform, and occasionally coalescent; moisture and trauma are important factors in promoting inoculation and rapid growth in the mucocutaneous genital areas.

Some warts resolve spontaneously within a few months, others persist for years, average duration being 2 years. Genital warts are often resistant to treatment and have a high relapse rate.

Problems

Diagnosis is usually easy.

Molluscum contagiosum can cause similar lesions, but tends to smooth pearly papules with umbilication. Periungual warts may be confused with the fibromata of epiloia. Plantar warts may be confused with corns and callosities which usually develop on pressure points, but on paring do not show capillary bleeding points. A wart is more painful on lateral pressure, and a callosity on direct pressure.

Plane warts may be confused with lichen planus, which tends to be more violaceous in colour and more irritant. Genital warts must be distinguished from condylomatalata, which are usually flatter and associated with other manifestations of secondary syphilis.

Apart from problems associated with diagnosis, decisions over treatment can be difficult. Painful or irritant warts must be dealt with, but with lesions that do not bother the patient, it may be difficult to decide whether to recommend treatments that may cause some discomfort, or whether it is wise to leave them alone, and allow spontaneous resolution. Time must be allowed to discuss the various options with either the patient himself, or the parents of affected children.

Assessment and investigation

Diagnosis is made on clinical grounds. If there is doubt, surface paring of a wart with a blade may show black specks, which are thrombosed capillaries, or bleeding points. Occasionally histology of curetted lesions may be required.

Management

Decisions over treatment depend on the number of lesions, discomfort, cosmetic status and the site of the lesions. Success of treatment depends on the cell-mediated immunity of the patient against the papova virus, and the method of treatment; multiple warts imply poor immunity, so radical treatments are not used for extensive and multiple lesions.

Caustics such as salicylic acid, trichloracetic acid and formalin are simple to use, and often effective when used correctly.

Podophyllin (25% in tinct. benz. co.) is more useful as weekly treatment for anogenital warts. (The podophyllin should be washed off after 6 hours.)

Liquid nitrogen cryotherapy is a popular treatment, and although this is generally available only through the hospital dermatology unit, there is no reason why it should not be made available in the general practice surgery, or on a domiciliary basis. Small lesions on thin skin should be treated for 10–15 seconds, and larger warts on thick skin for 30–60 seconds. Some may require local anaesthetic. A subepidermal blister forms in 2 days with the wart in the roof of the blister, the lesions disappearing with the blister over 2–3 weeks, cure being effected in about 80% of cases. However, curettage and cautery probably remain the most effective treatments for warts, despite the need for anaesthesia. The place of immunotherapy with vaccine remains to be seen.

2

FUNGAL INFECTIONS

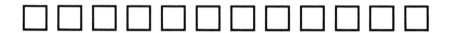

'RINGWORM' OR 'TINEA'

Introduction

These are vague terms for skin infections caused by *Trichophyton*, *Microsporum* and *Epidermophyton* fungi; a better collective term is 'dermatophyte infection'. These fungi inhabit and destroy keratin and some are able to live in hair or nails. Some cause annular, slowly outward-spreading lesions with central clearing which has given rise to the description 'ringworm'. *Tinea* is Latin for 'gnawing worm'.

The infection is contracted from infected skin fragments from humans and in some cases animals such as cats, dogs and cattle. The warmth and moisture of intertriginous skin is ideal for growth and survival of fungus and alteration of these conditions can be an important part of treatment. Infections of nails tend to persist and are difficult to treat.

Clinical features

Skin lesions tend to be erythematous and scaling, but not always in typical 'ring' form, and are occasionally macerated and irritating, fissured and painful, or vesicular (Figure 3) especially on the feet. Longstanding infections may become extensive and confluent, and occasionally there is a follicular, even pustular formation. Rarely a fungal folliculitis can become granulomatous.

Scalp infections, which are mostly limited to children, cause bald patches (Figure 4) and rarely an acute inflammatory response called a 'kerion'. A crust is formed over the scalp lesion in the condition favus, which is due to a specific *Trichophyton* sp. common in the Middle East.

Nail infections appear as a white or yellow discoloration at the side of the nail plate spreading to the base of the nail, but sometimes remaining in patches. The nail plate may thicken with cracking and lifting due to subungual hyperkeratosis, or it may become dystrophic and break off. Nail folds remain unaffected by ringworm infection.

Problems

Differential diagnosis may be difficult but, if there is doubt, skin scrapings, hairs and pieces of nail can easily be taken and sent to the hospital laboratory for mycological examination.

Clinically, eczema and psoriasis are mainly distinguished by symmetrical distribution and typical lesions elsewhere. Psoriasis tends to cause a well-demarcated patch rather than a confluent eruption. *Candida albicans* skin infections tend to have satellite lesions, and when infecting the nail plate, have associated swelling and redness of posterior nail fold. It must be remembered that not all deformed nails are the result of ringworm infection, but are frequently manifestations of eczema, psoriasis or lichen planus. Pitting of nails that occurs in psoriasis is not present in fungal infections.

Intertriginous erythrasma may cause confusion, but can be distinguished by a pink fluorescence under Wood's light.

Assessment and investigation

Diagnosis can usually be made on clinical grounds, and if necessary confirmed by mycological examination; the scrapings, nail pieces, or hairs are treated with potassium hydroxide to dissolve the keratin and then searched microscopically for hyphae. Culture, which takes 2–3 weeks, allows identification of the species of fungi.

Wood's filtered ultraviolet light is used mostly for diagnosis of fungal scalp infections, in which hairs will fluoresce bright green, and also for diagnosing erythrasma, when fluorescence is pink.

Management

The imidazole drugs – clotrimazole (Canesten), econazole (Ecostatin, Pevaryl) and miconazole (Daktarin, Dermonistat) – are the most effective topical antifungal agents, and have largely superseded Whitfield's ointment (benzoic acid 6% and salicylic acid 3%). The imidazoles also cover *Candida* and *Pityrosporum* organisms as well as ringworm, and resistance is not a problem. However, Whitfield's ointment is still very useful in some cases.

If there is a moist maceration of the rash, magenta paint lotion may be more effective and give greater symptomatic relief. In acute cases of infection of the feet, with blisters and exudation, potassium permanganate soaks 1:8000 for 15 minutes, four times a day, are often the best treatment.

Oral griseofulvin, which is active only against ringworm, tends to be more effective than topical agents in tinea cruris, manuum and corporis, and is generally taken in adult dosage of 500 mg daily for 1 month. In tinea capitis, griseofulvin is the only treatment that should be considered and is taken for 6 weeks. Griseofulvin is also usually required in nail infections and may be expected to clear fingernails in 3–6 months, but may need to be given for up to 2 years in toenail infections, and even then there is a relatively high incidence of reinfection.

If a toenail becomes so deformed as to interfere with the wearing of shoes, it should be avulsed. One technique is to apply 40% urea

15

in aqueous cream under an occlusive dressing for 10 days to soften the nail so that it can then be avulsed without requiring local anaesthesia.

Ketoconazole (Nizoral), the relatively new broad-spectrum antifungal, is effective against *Candida* spp. and pityriasis versicolor as well as all the ringworm infections. It is worth trying in nail infections, but like griseofulvin, tends to be disappointing in toenail infections. More experience in the use of ketoconazole needs to be gained; it can cause liver damage and is teratogenic to rats in high doses, so caution must be exercised. At present, it is most useful in severe cases of ringworm, such as scalp infection which requires a systemic drug, as a prophylactic against systemic candidiasis in immunosuppressed patients, and also in the rare mucocutaneous candidiasis.

CANDIDIASIS

Introduction

This is infection due to the ubiquitous *Candida albicans* fungus, which is essentially opportunistic in character, affecting previously traumatized skin or mucosa or occurring in the debilitated or those compromised by such conditions as diabetes, pregnancy and disturbance of the balance of normal flora of organisms such as occurs in antibiotic therapy.

Oral thrush and angular stomatitis occur in young infants, and in adults with previous oral disease or ill-fitting dentures, and in the debilitated. However, a chronic hyperplastic form of oral candidiosis is occasionally seen in middle-aged adults in whom no other abnormality is found, and manifests as white plaques.

Intertriginous and balanitic candidiases are usually secondary to moist maceration. Vulvovaginitis occasionally seems to be more spontaneous in nature, though diabetes, pregnancy, certain antibiotics and the contraceptive pill increase susceptibility, and some individuals appear to have an innate susceptibility to recurrent attacks for no good reason. Candidal paronychia is associated with moisture and is an occupational hazard in barmaids and fishmongers.

The serious disease of mucocutaneous candidiasis occurs in the immunologically compromised and may be associated with abnormality of endocrine function and iron deficiency. The granulomatous form occurs in children causing facial and scalp lesions, and the non-granulomatous form causes extensive lesions of the mouth and digits.

Clinical features

Skin lesions start as erythematous areas, with slight scaling at the edges with characteristically satellite papules and pustules. In advanced lesions, pustules appear within the confluent erythematous areas. There is usually pruritus. Mucosal lesions are typically creamy white plaques which are removed with difficulty to reveal a red base, although sometimes the lesions are merely inflamed erythematous areas with occasional ulcers.

Candidal paronychia is characterized by redness and swelling of posterior nail folds, early loss of cuticle, ridging of nail plate, and usually a brownish green discoloration. Pus is only slight, distinguishing the condition from bacterial paronychia.

Problems

Difficulties may occur in diagnosis, in discovering underlying conditions such as diabetes, and in modifying conditions to try and prevent recurrent infections in the susceptible.

The plaques of infant thrush must be distinguished from the more easily removed milk curds; in adults, if there are erosions, other causes may have to be considered, such as ill-fitting dentures, pemphigus, Behçet's disease and aphthous ulceration.

Intertriginous candidiasis may be confused with simple intertrigo, eczema, ringworm and erythrasma. Helpful pointers may be pustular satellite lesions and, in the final analysis, mycological study.

Diagnosis of genital candidiasis usually requires microscopy and culture of swabs, and, as well as searching for underlying disease such as diabetes, one should be alert for other associated genitourinary disease.

Assessment and investigation

Diagnosis is usually made on clinical grounds, but often confirmed by taking swabs for microscopy and culture, which are also helpful in revealing associated disease. Urinalysis for sugar is mandatory in assessment of these cases.

In paronychia, nail specimens may need to be taken in order to confirm diagnosis of *Candida* by mycological examination.

In recurrent or persistent cases, and especially in chronic mucocutaneous candidiasis, where a biopsy might be appropriate, tests of immunological competence should be performed; these include immunoglobulin assay, lymphocyte transformation by *Candida,* opsonizing function, and killing of *Candida* by phagocytes. Measurement of serum iron and tests of endocrine function might also be helpful in the assessment of this condition.

Management

Oral thrush in infants is usually treated with nystatin suspension, and in adults, sucking nystatin tablets or amphoteracin lozenges is generally more effective. For skin lesions, creams containing nystatin, miconazole or clotrimazole can be used although, if the skin is moist and weeping, magenta paint might be better. Some skin lesions – especially vulvitis and balanitis – are very irritant, and nystatin in combination with hydrocortisone cream is more helpful.

The most important aspect of treatment of chronic candidal paronychia is to keep the hands out of water and, if necessary, to wear cotton-lined rubber gloves, and if one is occupationally compromised to continue wearing them after the infection has cleared in order to prevent recurrence. Topical antifungal lotions applied to the junction of nail fold and nail plate may help slightly. It may take several months for paronychia to clear, and oral ketoconazole is useful in difficult cases.

Treatment of chronic mucocutaneous candidiasis involves correction of underlying abnormalities and giving ketaconazole, which has superseded amphoteracin therapy.

PITYRIASIS VERSICOLOR

Introduction

This is a worldwide infection caused by the fungus *Pityrosporum orbiculare*. It is more common in hot humid climates. The fungus produces a carboxylic acid which inhibits melanin formation causing loss of pigment, made obvious after exposure to sunlight.

Clinical features

The upper trunk is usually affected and the condition presents either as reddish brown scaly patches, or as hypopigmented areas which may coalesce. There is sometimes irritation. Rarely face and legs are affected.

Problems

Diagnosis is not usually a problem, but eczema, pityriasis rosea and erythrasma may cause confusion. When the patient presents with hypopigmented areas, vitiligo has to be considered. Pigmentation may not return for several months after treatment. Certain individuals seem to be prone to persistent and recurrent infection.

Assessment and investigation

Diagnosis is usually on clinical grounds, but can be confirmed by direct microscopy which usually demonstrates numerous spores in addition to the hyphae. Culture is difficult.

Treatment

Half-strength Whitfield's ointment, clotrimazole (Canesten), miconazole (Daktarin), and 20% sodium thiosulphate solution can all be used. Application is nightly to the whole trunk for a month. The shampoo Selsun (selenium sulphide 2.5% suspension) is also useful, being left on overnight, and this may be combined with a morning application of one of the above ointments or creams. Oral ketoconazole (Nizoral) 200 mg daily for 2 weeks is also effective, and is the only systemic treatment available.

3

BACTERIAL INFECTIONS

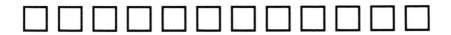

IMPETIGO

Introduction

This is one of the commonest infections, especially in children, and it is often misdiagnosed. The usual cause is *Staphylococcus aureus,* but the haemolytic streptococcus may also be present in the infected area, and it is important to remember that cardiac and renal complications, which may follow infection with this organism, typically in the upper respiratory tract, may also follow an infection in the skin.

Impetigo is an infection of the epidermis; the initial lesions usually manifest as thin-roofed purulent blisters which rupture to form superficial erosions (Figure 5). The lesions may form crusts made up of keratin, serous exudate and pus. Erosions tend to coalesce and satellite lesions are common. The hands and face are the commonest sites for impetigo due to ease of spread from one area to the other.

Problems and management

Diagnosis may be difficult and, in the absence of typical lesions, a helpful pointer is the asymmetry of the eruption as distinct from an endogenous eczema.

Assessment may be made more difficult because of prior use of topical steroids which reduce crusting and the typical golden appearance of the lesions.

A further problem is that impetigo may be secondary to other skin diseases such as eczema, and in these circumstances the clinical picture may be confusing and the infection may extend beyond the epidermis, necessitating the use of systemic antibiotics and follow-up for later treatment of the underlying condition.

Impetigo is a contagious disorder and mothers of affected children must be advised over personal hygiene and keeping the child away from school. It may be wise to take swabs from the nostrils of the patient and other members of the family, as the offending organisms are often harboured in the anterior nares where they can be eradicated quite easily by topical antibiotics.

For actual treatment of the lesions it is important that the crusts are removed by soap and water before application of topical antibiotics, in order to facilitate adequate penetration of the drug. Systemic antibiotics (flucloxacillin or erythromycin) are generally used only when the condition is very extensive. Topical antibiotics commonly used are fusidic acid and neomycin.

ECTHYMA

This is a deeper version of impetigo, the erosion extending into the upper dermis to form a shallow ulcer with an adherent crust. Healing leaves a superficial scar. The lesion may be solitary and occurs most commonly on the lower legs, perhaps following minor trauma. Poor hygiene and neglect are other predisposing factors. Systemic antibiotics in addition to topical antibiotics are required for treatment, as there is involvement of the dermis.

FOLLICULITIS

This is an inflammation in the opening of the hair follicles, manifest clinically as discrete small pustules which heal without scarring. The condition can be caused by (1) bacterial infection, (2) chemical irritation such as that resulting from contact with certain oils and (3) physical damage, such as occurs in the beard area when short curling hairs grow back into the skin. (4) Folliculitis may also occur as a manifestation of seborrhoeic eczema. The treatment of the folliculitis will depend on the cause. If it is due to bacterial infection, antibiotics – topical and/or systemic – are necessary. It is also important to treat the staphylococcal carrier sites with topical antibiotics in persistent or recurrent folliculitis. If the folliculitis is due to oils and grease, removal of the offending substances, and simple keratolytics, e.g. 2% salicylic acid lotion or cream, will speed resolution. In cases of folliculitis due to seborrhoeic eczema treatment as for eczema is required.

FURUNCULOSIS

This is a staphylococcal infection of the hair follicle that spreads into the dermis forming a 'boil'. Clinically the lesion begins as a small red nodule which increases in size and becomes fluctuant with 2–3 days. The lesion is firmly contained in the dermis and the apex gradually 'points' and then breaks down to discharge pus and necrotic tissue, and eventually heals leaving a small scar.

A carbuncle is a coalescent aggregation of a number of furuncles. Sycosis is a chronic/subacute staphylococcal infection of the hair follicles commonly affecting the beard area, but also occurring in scalp, axillae and genital areas; the condition lies somewhere between a folliculitis and a furunculosis.

It is important to investigate patients with recurrent staphylococcal skin infections for possible predisposing factors such as diabetes, malabsorption and reticulosis, as a 'boil' may be the first sign of the underlying condition. The commonest cause of recurrent boils is harbouring of the staphylococcus in the anterior nares, axillae or perineum, and swabs should be taken from these sites and appropriate topical antibiotics applied twice daily for at least 1 month if the organism is found. Systemic antibiotics are indicated in large boils and carbuncles. Incision to drain pus may also be necessary.

ERYSIPELAS

This is a streptococcal cellulitis that may affect any area but typically occurs on the face and scalp, the organism gaining entry through a small crack in the skin or the nostril or external auditory canal, or via breaks in the skin caused by other dermatoses such as eczema. Clinically the cellulitis is red, hot and indurated, and has a distinct border which may be vesiculated. The condition can be severe with marked constitutional upset, and systemic (sometimes intravenous) antibiotics, usually flucloxacillin or erythromycin as first line drugs, are required for treatment.

TUBERCULOUS SKIN INFECTION

This is now rare. Lupus vulgaris is the commonest type of lesion usually occurring on the hands or the neck, and presenting as a chronic reddish nodular plaque which if pressed with a glass spatula exhibits the typical brownish 'apple-jelly nodules'. The infiltrated plaque invades the dermis leading to scarring. Tuberculous verrucosa cutis is a granulomatous skin lesion resulting from direct inoculation of tubercle bacilli, and scrofuloderma is an extension of tuberculous infection to the skin from an underlying focus in bones or lymph nodes.

The treatment of skin tuberculosis is the same as for tuberculosis elsewhere, with various appropriate combinations of rifampicin, streptomycin, isoniazid and ethambutol.

SYPHILIS

The primary lesion, or chancre, is a small nodule which quickly breaks down to form a painless ulcer with a red indurated border usually less than 1 cm in diameter. There may be associated regional lymphadenopathy. The ulcer usually heals in 3–6 weeks leaving an atrophic scar.

The rash of secondary syphilis may appear within 6 weeks and up to 1 year after initial infection and may be difficult to diagnose as it often resembles other dermatoses, particularly guttate psoriasis and pityriasis rosea. The eruption varies in type and extent, and may be macular, papular, papulosquamous (i.e. scaly) or pustular; the lesions may start as discrete pink papules but they can merge to form a confluent scaly dermatosis. The condition often affects the palms, and if it is seen in the papular and not the squamous form this acts as a diagnostic pointer, because this type of palmar eruption does not occur in eczema, psoriasis or pityriasis rosea.

In moist areas around the genitalia and perianal skin the papules become hypertrophic, eroded and exudative, and are known as condylomata lata; these may be difficult to distinguish from viral warts.

On the mucous membranes, lesions occur as smooth nodules or grey patches, both tending to ulcerate, giving rise to the classical snail track ulcers.

Patchy hair loss may occur in secondary syphilis and is characteristically incomplete or 'moth-eaten'.

Skin manifestations of tertiary syphilis consist of (1) irregular, scaly, reddish brown nodules, (2) gummata, which are masses of syphilitic granulation tissue which break through the skin to form slow growing painless ulcers, and (3) chronic interstitial glossitis appearing as extensive irregular fissuring with accompanying leukoplakia.

In the management of syphilis, contact tracing is most important. Penicillin is the drug of choice given by intramuscular injection. Aqueous procaine penicillin is given for the primary and secondary stages, 600 000 units daily for 10 days for the former and for 2 weeks for the latter. In tertiary syphilis 12 megaunits of procaine penicillin should be given over a period of 3 weeks. If patients are allergic to penicillin, erythromycin or tetracycline, 30 g over a period of 2 weeks, should be prescribed.

ERYTHRASMA

This is caused by the bacterium *Corynebacterium minutissimum*. The sites affected are the intertriginous areas, i.e. axillae, groins, peri-anal skin and between the toes. The lesions present as reddish-brown (Figure 6) scaly patches. The lesions may be asymptomatic or cause mild irritation. They respond to oral tetracycline and erythromycin, or topical sodium fusidate (Fucidin) ointment.

4

TROPICAL INFECTIONS

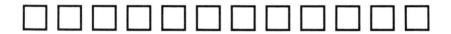

Tropical infections are rarely seen in the United Kingdom, but because of the immigrant population and the increasing number of people travelling abroad, both on business and on holiday, it has become important to acquire a greater awareness of at least some of the commoner tropical dermatoses such as leprosy, yaws, and leishmaniasis.

LEPROSY

This occurs throughout the tropics but is more common in West Africa, India and the Far East. The condition affects all races and has an incubation period of between 2 and 5 years. The disease varies in severity according to the patient's resistance to *Mycobacterium leprae*. In 'lepromatous' leprosy there is little immunity, and the lesions, which contain many organisms, are progressive and destructive. In 'tuberculoid' leprosy resistance is high, organisms rare, and the course of the disease is benign with a tendency to spontaneous cure; lesions present as infiltrated plaques, often hypopigmented, anaesthetic and hypohydrotic. The neuropathy of leprosy may lead to trophic and traumatic changes in the skin.

Treatment regimes depend on the type of leprosy. The drugs most commonly used are rifampicin and dapsone.

YAWS

This is caused by the spirochaete *Treponema pertenue,* and is common in the West Indies. The primary lesion, which develops 3–4 weeks after inoculation, is a solitary papule which enlarges and satellite lesions occur which becomes confluent and crusted. Two to 3 months later the secondary stage occurs which is a papular or granulomatous eruption: these lesions may persist for several months but then fade without scarring. Tertiary yaws occurs a few years later and most commonly affects the skin and bones. Spreading ulcers of the skin may lead to severe scarring. Granulomatous nodules, periostitis, tenosynovitis and hyperkeratosis of palms and soles may occur. In yaws, unlike syphilis, the cardiovascular and nervous systems are not involved. Treatment is with penicillin.

CUTANEOUS LEISHMANIASIS

This is caused by a protozoon transmitted by the sandfly. The disease occurs in the Middle East, Southern Mediterranean, Africa, Asia and Central and South America. The incubation period may extend to several months before the typical skin lesions appear and they are sited usually on the exposed areas. Initially there is a small papule; this enlarges to form a nodule or plaque, later becoming scaly and ulcerated, so forming the 'Oriental Sore' (Figure 7). Diagnosis is made by detecting Leishman–Donovan bodies in smears of the ulcer, and occasionally by biopsy and culture. The lesion usually heals after a few months leaving a depressed scar. Some cases may by persistent and slow to improve and treatment can then be effected with intralesional and systemic steroids combined with injections of organic antimony.

5

PARASITIC INFESTATIONS

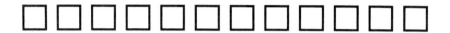

SCABIES

Introduction

Scabies is a contagious infestation of the skin by an insect, or mite, called *Sarcoptes scabei* var. *hominis*. The female mite (acarus) burrows into the keratin layer of the epidermis to lay her eggs, which, on hatching, produce an intensely irritating eruption, usually worse at night.

Clinical features

The burrows of the acarus may be seen as greyish, linear, or slightly curved scaly lesions up to 1 cm long, commonly on wrists and palms and in the webs between fingers. Other lesions seen are superficial, scaly and often excoriated areas which may become crusted or pustular due to secondary infection. Also, firm, deep, red papules may occur especially in male patients on the buttocks and genitalia.

The eruption may become generalized as excoriated papular urticarial lesions extending over limbs and trunk (Figure 8), but never above the neck except in the case of children under the age of 2 years. Lesions in children are usually firm red papules particularly in and around the axillae, although under the age of 1 year a common site for burrows is the soles of the feet where they may present as small blisters.

Problems

Because of excoriations, possible secondary infection and impetigo, nodular and urticarial allergic reactions to the mite and its products, the primary condition may be difficult to recognize. If there is any suspicion of the infestation a thorough search for the acarus can be carried out by gently scraping a papule, or what is thought to be a burrow, with a blunt scalpel blade and examining the contents under a low power microscope field. However, in most circumstances, diagnosis is made and treatment instituted merely on clinical appearances, and sometimes only on a high index of suspicion without definite diagnosis.

Other problems with scabies may derive from (1) inefficient treatment, (2) failure to treat close contact family and friends and (3) ignorance over the fact that irritation may persist for 2 weeks after treatment, and that papular lesions, especially in children, may persist for many months after treatment, both being allergic phenomena which sometimes lead to needless overtreatment and occasionally an iatrogenic eczema.

Management

Benzyl benzoate application B.P. 25% and gamma benzene hexa-chloride lotion 1% or cream are commonly used treatments. The usual method is to have a bath, dry, and then apply the preparation with cotton wool to *all* the skin surface from the neck to the soles of the feet, and leave for 24 hours, after which the sequence is repeated for the second and final time. Close contacts should be treated simultaneously. Crotamiton lotion can be useful in control-ling the itching that persists after treatment.

Bedsheets and underwear should be changed, but it is not necessary to clean outer garments or blankets.

PEDICULOSIS (LICE)

Head lice are common in children , causing irritation, excoriation and secondary impetigo. The condition is usually recognized by the presence of 'nits' which are seen as small white specks and distinguished from seborrhoeic eczema scales by their firm attachment to the hair shaft. Common treatments are gamma benzene hexachloride solution 1%, malathion 0.5%, and carbaryl 0.5% lotion, the former being applied to washed hair and left for 24 hours, and the latter two preparations being applied to dry hair and left for 12 hours. After the said interval the hair is shampooed and combed through with a fine comb while wet. The treatment is repeated after a week. It is probably advisable to treat all members of the family, especially children, at the same time, even if they have no symptoms.

Body lice are rare, being associated with very poor personal hygiene such as occurs in tramps, the louse actually living in the underclothing, where it may be visible to the naked eye; bites are commonly on the trunk and cause small red macules and papules with central haemorrhagic punctum, although, owing to severe itching, the lesions may be camouflaged by severe excoriations, secondary infection, eczema and lichenification, and various pigmentary changes; when all of these secondary effects are present, the condition is known as 'vagabond's disease'. For treatment, 1% gamma-benzene-hexachloride cream is applied to the body, while clothes are treated with the same compound in lotion or power form and then sent for laundering.

Pubic lice produce irritation, excoriations and secondary problems in a similar way, and the condition can also affect axillary hair, eyelashes and eyebrows. Treatment is as for head lice.

31

INSECT BITES

The bites of fleas, flies, mosquitoes, bedbugs and other insects usually cause a relatively mild, but often very itchy, urticarial lesion with central punctum and surrounding flare, the spots usually occurring in groups, asymmetrically, on exposed parts. However, the clinical picture may vary in two ways: (1) the initial urticarial reaction may be much more acute, with formation of blisters and (2) the initial lesion may not fade over the usual 2–3 days, but instead form persistent papules which are itchy and may take months to clear. In Negroes, this type of papular urticaria invariably leads to postinflammatory hyperpigmentation.

Treatment

Mild and moderate reactions are treated by cleansing, and applying a cooling lotion such as calamine, and giving oral antihistamines to reduce irritation. Active infestation can be treated effectively with applications such as monosulfiram solution.

Very acute blistering eruptions require systemic antihistamines and possibly a short course of systemic steroids, with careful dressings to prevent secondary infection. Bee stings should be scraped off with a fingernail or knife before dressing the area. Anaphylactic reactions require treatment with subcutaneous or intramuscular adrenaline, probably in conjunction with intravenous steroids and antihistamines, although mild reactions can be treated with adrenaline inhalation (1–3 puffs of Medihaler-epi) and it is sensible for patients at risk to keep such an inhaler at the ready.

One of the problems in treating papular urticaria is to convince the patient or parent of the aetiology, and to explain that the lesion is due more to an altered immunological response than to the insect bite itself. Fortunately most children seem to lose this hypersensitivity response to insect bites in due course. If the source of the problem is identified it should be treated and in the case of a domestic pet it may be helpful to confer with the vet. Furniture may harbour insects and this can be treated effectively with powders containing pyrethrum. For the patient with papular urticaria due to insect bites antihistamines once again provide the mainstay of therapy.

6

ECZEMA

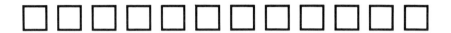

'Eczema' is used synonomously with 'dermatitis', which is a commoner term in American texts. Eczema denotes a particular inflammatory reaction in the skin which appears to have a number of different causes although the final pathogenic events are similar.

There are two major groups of eczema, namely that which is produced by external substances, exogenous eczema, and that which appears to be due to internal or constitutional factors, termed endogenous eczema. It is important to distinguish between these two groups of eczema, for in exogenous eczema identifying the causative agent may result in a permanent cure, whilst in endogenous eczema the treatment is suppressive rather than curative.

EXOGENOUS ECZEMA

Exogenous eczema may be due to two groups of substances, namely primary irritants and allergens.

Primary irritant eczema

Introduction

Irritants are chemicals which directly damage the skin, particularly the keratin which acts as a protective barrier. Once the protective function of the keratin is impaired irritant chemicals are able to pass into the cellular component of the epidermis and cause an inflammatory reaction. The chemicals causing irritant eczema are common substances both in the home and at work. In the home they include detergents, cleansers, bleaches, washing powders, soaps and solvents. At work the common ones are cutting oils, acids, alkalis and solvents. Continual wetting of the skin – e.g. in barworkers and fishmongers who do not dry the skin – will lead to evaporation of water and cooling of the skin which results in cracking of the keratin and allows penetration of irritant substances. A similar effect is seen in children who dribble a great deal, and develop an irritant eczema around the mouth. It seems that there are constitutional factors which predispose to the development of irritant eczema as certain individuals appear more prone than others, although exposure to the same substances is similar.

Clinical features

The commonest site of irritant eczema is the hands, as they are the part of the body more likely to be in contact with irritants. Weak irritants which are common in the home cause dryness and scaling with superficial cracking. After long-term use there is redness and fissuring. The backs of the hands, web spaces and backs of the fingers show these features before the palms, where the keratin is thinner. When there is contact with strong irritants, there is erythema, and vesiculation which may break down to form superficial ulcers and crusts.

Assessment and investigation

When the features suggest an exogenous eczema, it is important to decide whether patients are allergic to a particular substance or if it is an irritant, and patch tests may be necessary. If substances are thought to be primary irritants they should be diluted prior to testing, otherwise severe reactions may occur. In addition, if the substances are diluted sufficiently then no reaction will occur, whereas if the substance is a true allergen then patients will still react despite dilution.

Management

Patients should be advised to wear protective clothing to keep the substances away from the skin. Rubber gloves are usually sufficient in the home, and the gloves should preferably have a cotton lining, or patients should wear cotton gloves inside the rubber ones. It is sometimes difficult for patients to carry out intricate tasks on machinery with gloves, but they should be encouraged to do so. Changing the job should be the last resort. Washing off the irritant chemicals as soon as possible is important. Barrier creams help but they are not as effective as gloves. If cold weather and moisture are aggravating factors keeping the hands warm with gloves and the use of emollients is helpful.

If the eczema is severe, with vesiculation and crusts, then the hands should be soaked in potassium permanganate solution 1:8000, three times a day for 15 minutes each time. When the eczema is dry and scaly, topical steroid ointments should be used to clear the eczema.

Secondary infection is a complication of any eczema and if it occurs antibiotics should be given.

Referral to specialist. This is only necessary if the condition does not clear with the above measures, or if it is considered necessary to carry out patch tests.

Long-term care. If patients are prone to develop irritant eczema then that tendency will probably persist for life. Nevertheless, if the exposure to the irritants can be stopped or at least decreased the eventual outlook is good. It does seem, however, that in certain individuals, that once eczema develops it may be some time before it is controlled despite no further contact with irritants.

Allergic contact eczema

Introduction

This is caused by the skin becoming sensitized to a specific antigen, which on further exposure results in an inflammatory reaction in the skin. Why some patients develop sensitivity to certain chemicals and others do not is unknown. Once patients develop this sensitivity it tends to last indefinitely.

There are numerous chemicals which may sensitize patients. A number of these substances are very common, e.g. dyes in clothing, or nickel in jewellery and watch straps, whilst others are rare and tend to be found only in certain industrial processes, so only those subjects who come into contact with them at work will be at risk. The common contact allergens are listed in Table 6.1.

Table 6.1   Common contact allergens

Substance	Source
Allergens	
Nickel	Jewellery, zips, underwear fasteners, metal buttons, watch straps
Cobalt	Cement Some printing inks
Chromates	Cement, leather, matches
Rubber	Elastic, shoes
Dyes	Hair dyes, clothing
Lanolin	Cosmetics, ointments
Colophony	Sticking plasters, soaps
Balsams (from plants) and synthetic volatile oils	Perfumes
Formaldehyde	Plastics, cosmetics, glues
Epoxy resin	Glues, do-it-yourself hardeners
Phosphorus sesquisulphide	Matches
Sulphonamide–formaldehyde polymer resin	Nail varnish
Plants	Primula, poison ivy
Applied medicaments	
Antibiotics (neomycin, soframycin)	Antibiotic creams
Antihistamines	Anti-itch creams
Antiseptics (chlorhexidine, chloroxylenol)	Dettol, Germolene, Savlon, Hibitane
Local anaesthetics	Pain and itch relieving creams
Preservatives	Creams, lotions and ointments

Clinical features

Contact allergic eczema is rare before the age of 15 and in the elderly, and this may be related to impaired cell-mediated immunity in the elderly.

The site and pattern of the eczema depends on site of contact; however, the penetration of the allergen will be more rapid through thin and moist skin. Thus when the face is exposed to an allergen the eczema will first appear around the eyes, where the skin is thinnest on the face. Contact to the dye in tights may appear in the popliteal fossae where the skin is thinnest on the legs, or on the feet due to hydration of the keratin from sweating. Contact eczema on the hands will appear on the back of the hands and web spaces before the palms. The site of the eczema may well suggest the allergen; e.g. ear lobes – suggests nickel allergy from ear-rings; apex of the axillae – perfumes in deodorants; hands and lower forearms – rubber from rubber gloves. However, the nature of the allergen is not always obvious; thus eczema on the face may be due to a substance in cosmetics, or in smoke from the phosphorus sesquisulphide in matches, or from nail varnish (Figure 9). Sometimes the cause of the allergen is unexpected, e.g. contact eczema on a man's face due to his wife's perfume.

Contact eczema is often suggested by a sharp cut-off point between the affected and unaffected skin, the eczema only occurring at the exact sites of contact. Allergic contact eczema is often acute with intense erythema, weeping and vesiculation. However, there are variations in presentation of contact eczema, in that the eczema may spread beyond and around the site of contact. In addition allergens which are absorbed into the circulation on the sensitized lymphocytes travel to other parts of the body where eczema may appear without direct contact. This is most commonly seen with nickel, in that the eczema often appears in the antecubital fossae and around the eyes. Finally it must be remembered that any eczema may spread to other sites in a non-specific pattern, due to so-called autosensitization, and this occurs both with endogenous and exogenous eczema.

Problems

It is often not appreciated by patients that contact eczema may occur after only two exposures to the allergen or after several years of exposure. Patients feel that if they have used a substance for several years without trouble, it is unlikely to be the cause of the eczema.

The differential diagnosis of contact allergic eczema is most commonly from other forms of eczema, and will depend on the site. On the hands irritant eczema and endogenous hand eczema have to be considered. On the feet, endogenous eczema and fungal infections are the common differential diagnoses. On the face, particularly around the eyes, seborrhoeic or atopic eczema may give similar appearances.

Assessment and investigation

Allergic contact eczema is established by so-called *patch tests*. In this procedure the suspected substance is applied to the skin under an occlusive dressing for 48h. If the patient is allergic to the substance a patch of eczema will be present at the patch test site. Occasionally, however, there is a delayed reaction and the site should be inspected again after a further 48h. It is important to know that some substances which may act as irritants or are strong sensitizers should be diluted before being applied and occluded. If the cause of the eczema is obvious – e.g. acute eczema on the face and scalp after using a hair dye – then patch tests may not be necessary.

Management

If the eczema is severe with exudation, normal saline or potassium permanganate 1:8000 soaks or compresses should be used. Soaks are only convenient for hands and feet. The soaks or compresses should be carried out three or four times a day. Weak topical steroid creams should be applied four times a day. If the eczema is chronic and dry, potent topical steroid ointments may be used except for the face and intertriginous areas. If the eczema is very severe and widespread, a short course of systemic steroids, starting at 30mg daily of prednisone, should be prescribed.

Referral to specialist. This is only necessary if the allergen is not apparent and the eczema persists. Removal of the allergen will result in a cure. If the allergen is encountered at work, it will probably be necessary for the patient to be removed from the allergen's source. Unlike the effect of irritants, contact with even small quantities of the allergen may cause severe eczema.

ENDOGENOUS ECZEMA

This specific form of skin inflammation occurs in constitutionally predisposed individuals. External factors may exacerbate the condition, but are not causative. It is best to split the endogenous eczemas into the following types:

(1)   Atopic
(2)   Seborrhoeic
(3)   Discoid
(4)   Pompholyx
(5)   Lichen simplex
(6)   Asteatotic
(7)   Hypostatic

Atopic eczema

Introduction

This is sometimes called 'infantile' eczema because of the usual time of onset, between ages 2 and 12 months. About 25% of the population are potentially atopic, that is, have a genetically determined predisposition to atopic eczema, asthma, rhinitis and conjunctivitis; only 5% of these individuals will actually develop atopic eczema. Ninety per cent of cases clear by the age of 12, but 10% recur during teenage years; most are clear by 30 years.

Although genetic factors are important in atopic eczema the pathogenetic pathways are not known, but two possible hypotheses have been put forward: (1) deficiency of intestinal mucosal IgA and (2) deficiency of T-suppressor cells in early infancy. In both cases overproduction of IgE occurs in response to excess untrapped antigen. Breastfeeding is thought to be helpful in preventing eczema by supplying antibody to 'mop up' this excess antigen.

Clinical features

The infantile eruption is symmetrical, affecting face and trunk, but in early childhood the eczema takes on the typical flexural distribution, although in Negro children it is common to see the 'reverse' extensor pattern; late onset, 'extensor' pattern, associated asthma, family and social problems are all bad prognostic indicators.

Typically lesions are red and scaly, with weeping when acute, or crusting when subacute, and thickened scaly skin when chronic. Small red papules are common and vesicles are rare. Pruritus is intense and leads to excoriations (Figure 10). Repeated scratching causes lichenification and later excoriated papules and nodules. Postinflammatory hypo- and hyperpigmentation are common.

The condition can be aggravated by cold and occasionally by hot, humid conditions, also by wool, cosmetics, infections and emotional stress.

Secondary infection of eczema with staphylococci or streptococci is a common problem. Children with atopic eczema are more likely to develop viral problems such as warts and molluscum contagiosum, and herpes simplex infections may disseminate to give rise to Kaposi's varicelliform eruption.

Problems

Diagnosis is usually straightforward, but some cases of seborrhoeic and contact eczema may cause confusion; distribution of the eruption and family history often provide the key.

43

Treatment of mild cases may be easy, and 90% of eczema remits in childhood, but severe cases or chronic cases can be very difficult to treat and, in addition to exacting therapy, time must be spent with the parents in order to discuss the nature of the condition and give advice, reassurance and encouragement.

Eczema is exacerbated by emotional stress, and an attack of eczema, possibly accompanied by another manifestation of atopy such as asthma, in turn creates distress thus setting up a vicious circle which is often difficult to break; counselling and helping with social problems may be more useful than drugs.

Management

All treatment aims at keeping the skin as supple as possible. Emollients such as oilatum oil and emulsifying ointment should be added to bathing water, and soap avoided. After baths, and at other times, emollients such as E.45 or aqueous cream should be applied. All these preparations act by (1) soothing and (2) increasing hydration of stratum corneum by reducing water lost in evaporation.

Topical steroids provide the most effective treatment. The strength, quantity and type of application depend on the severity of the eczema and the type of skin affected. The weakest dilution possible should be used in order to avoid the complications of local thinning of skin and erythema, and possible systemic effects of absorbed steroids causing adrenal suppression and stunting of growth in children.

For the delicate skin of the face one rarely needs a stronger preparation than 1% hydrocortisone cream, whereas for thick lichenified patches of eczema on the limbs, full-strength potent topical steroid applications such as clobetasol propionate (Dermovate) may be used. Following improvement with steroids, withdrawal should be gradual with stepwise reduction in strength of application in order to prevent recurrence. As a general rule very potent topical steroids should only be used for 2-week periods at a time, which is usually sufficient to clear most atopic eczema. The very potent topical steroids may be used every 2 months, and at this frequency are usually safe. They should not be used in the intertriginous areas or on the face.

Crude coal tar is effective in eczema and may be used as a topical application but is best used mixed with emulsifying ointment (20% liquor picis carb. in emulsifying ointment) as a soap substitute. Coal tar impregnated bandages are useful for the legs.

It is important to treat pruritus in order to reduce distress as well as prevent excoriations and lichenification, and oral antihistamines are used, mostly at nights, when their sedative effect is probably more important than their antipruritic effect. Trimeprazine is a popular antihistamine and more recently ketotifen has been claimed to be useful.

Sudden temperature changes and exposure to cold winds should be avoided because of drying and cracking effects. Wool and manmade fibres should also be avoided, and stress minimized. Evidence that special diets may help in some cases is not yet clear but, needless to say, some parents are adamant that low allergen diet with exclusion of milk causes an improvement in their children's eczema. Breastfeeding seems to reduce the incidence of eczema in the first year, but long-term effects are not yet known. Recently, a well-controlled trial has shown some improvement in patients taking evening primrose oil.

Seborrhoeic eczema

Introduction

This is a characteristically scaly eczema affecting areas rich in sebaceous glands, or intertriginous areas, mostly scalp, alinasal folds, and flexures. The two distinct clinical types are (1) infantile (consisting mainly of 'cradle cap' and 'nappy rash') and (2) adult type in which dandruff and intertrigo are often mild manifestations.

Clinical features

Infantile type starts earlier than atopic eczema, often in the first month and mostly within 3 months. 'Cradle cap' scales may be fine and white, or thick and greasy. 'Napkin rash' might only be a moist maceration, but elsewhere shows 'psoriasiform' scaling. Face, neck, axillae, trunk, elbow and knee flexures may be affected (Figure 11). Pruritus is not a feature. Most children are clear by 18 months and the condition does not predispose to adult seborrhoeic eczema.

The adult type commences from the teens upwards. Scalp, periorbital and auricular areas, and nasolabial folds (Figure 12) are commonly affected. Forehead, cheeks (Figure 13), centres of chest and back, and all intertriginous areas (Figure 14) can be affected, with severe cases becoming generalized. There is erythema and scaling which may be fine and white or thick and yellow, occasionally becoming crusted with weeping and rarely with perifollicular pustules. The condition is often very itchy, and made worse by stress and fatigue. Sunlight may help. The course of the eczema is very chronic with relapses and remissions, and different areas being affected at different times.

Problems

At first sight, cradle cap may be very alarming to the parent, but fortunately treatment is simple and reassurance straightforward. A common problem with nappy rash is secondary infection with *Candida* which may give rise to satellite erythematous and pustular lesions.

Occasionally atopic eczema may be difficult to distinguish from infantile seborrhoeic eczema, but family history, late onset, different distribution and pruritus usually provide the answer, and this is important in relation to discussing prognosis with the parent.

Adult seborrhoeic eczema of scalp and intertriginous areas, when severe, may be confused with psoriasis. In the groins it may be confused with a fungal infection. When eyelids alone are involved, a contact eczema should be excluded.

Assessment and investigation

In many cases, swabs for bacteriology and mycology are required either for initial assessment, or for diagnosis of secondary infection. In addition, scrapings can be examined for fungus. If a contact eczema is suspected, patch testing should be carried out.

Management

Cradle cap is easily treated with a mild keratolytic such as 1% sulphur and 1% salicylic acid in aqueous cream, applying in the evening two or three times per week with shampooing next morning; for mild cases simple applications such as olive oil may suffice.

Infantile seborrhoeic eczema of trunk and nappy area should be treated by a mild steroid such as 1% hydrocortisone, combined with nystatin in the nappy area if *Candida* is suspected. Emulsifying ointment should be used as a soap substitute. Diapers should be changed regularly and left off for several hours each day.

In the adult the scalp is treated in a similar way, but with stronger keratolytics; up to 5% strength sulphur and salicylic acid creams and ung. cocois co. are commonly used. If scaling and irritation are severe, potent steroid lotion can be applied between hair washes.

Weak steroids are used for seborrhoeic eczema of the face, while trunk and intertriginous areas require moderate strength steroids. Antiseptic paints such as 1% aqueous gentian violet or magenta paint can be useful in intertriginous areas as they are drying and prevent secondary infection, and topical steroids can be applied after drying of the paint.

Discoid eczema

Introduction

Otherwise known as nummular eczema, this is characterized by well-defined coin-like lesions distributed symmetrically on extensor surfaces of the limbs and dorsal aspects of hands and feet. It may be associated with pompholyx eczema.

47

Clinical features

The lesions are scaly plaques (Figure 15), and if acute may have vesicles and exude serum. They are often very itchy. The condition can occur at any age, but it is most common between the ages of 20 and 40. As well as limbs, hands and feet, nail folds can be affected causing nail ridging, and rarely the face is affected. Despite a good response to treatment, relapses tend to occur.

Problems

A few lesions may resemble tinea, but lack of central clearing and negative mycology usually define the condition.

Lichen simplex is distinguished by more solitary and lichenified lesions. Plaques of mycosis fungoides can resemble discoid eczema, but they are persistent. A biopsy may have to be taken for confirmation.

Management

Lesions usually respond to moderate strength steroids, but occasionally potent steroid applications are required. Antihistamines may be required for pruritus in the early stages before the eczema clears with topical steroids.

Pompholyx eczema

Introduction

This is one of the most incapacitating eczemas, being localized to palms and soles and characterized by very itchy vesicles and bullae, and painful fissures.

The condition may be associated with excess sweating, discoid eczema, nickel sensitivity and fungal infection. In nickel-sensitive subjects it has been claimed that exacerbation may be related to a recent high intake of nickel such as occurs in eating acidic fruit boiled in stainless steel saucepans (which contain small amounts of nickel).

Clinical features

Usually presenting in young adults, the eruption is commonly symmetrical and begins in the emotional sweat areas, i.e. palms, soles, and sides and dorsum of digits. As in other types of eczema, in severe cases eruptions may be spread to backs of hands and feet, and to the limbs.

The initial small itchy vesicles (Figure 16) may expand and coalesce to form bullae. These may dry up or persist and occasionally become secondarily infected and lead to cellulitis. In chronic pompholyx, palms and soles become dry and scaly with painful fissures, and nails become ridged if nail folds are involved. Attacks of pompholyx may be precipitated by heat or emotion, presumably mediated by excessive sweating.

Problems

A common difficulty is to differentiate from localized pustular psoriasis which tends to be less itchy and more clearly demarcated. Vesicles may occur with an acute fungal infection. Chronic dry scaly pompholyx may be confused with irritant and atopic eczema, psoriasis or fungal infections, the clue to diagnosis usually being provided by lesions elsewhere. Swabs and scrapings may have to be taken for analysis.

Management

Acute blistering pompholyx is best treated by potassium permanganate soaks 1:8000 for 15 minutes, three times daily. After drying, a weak steroid is applied.

The dry cracking chronic stage requires moderate to strong steroid applications. Emollients such as 20% liquor picis carb. in emulsifying ointment may also be helpful. Tinct. benz. co. is helpful for fissures.

Systemic steroids may be required in severe attacks, antibiotics for secondary infection and antihistamines for pruritus.

Lichen simplex

Introduction

This can be regarded as a localized form of atopic eczema. It occurs mainly in adults, women more commonly than men, and there is often other personal or family history of atopy.

Clinical features

The lesions are solitary, sited typically at nape of neck, and less commonly on forearms, wrists, shins and ankles. Variable-size plaques are formed and itching is intense. Lichenification with exaggerated skin ridges occurs, and the lesions are often reddish purple and hyperpigmented. Scratching tends to perpetuate the lesion, and recurrence is common, with permanent resolution usually occurring in old age.

Problems

Single lesion discoid eczema may cause diagnostic confusion but lichenification is absent. Hypertrophic lichen planus on the legs is distinguished by the purple colour. Lichen amyloid on the lower limbs may be very itchy, but its symmetrical distribution and rippled appearance differentiate it from lichen simplex. Skin biopsy is occasionally required to confirm a diagnosis of lichen simplex.

Treatment

Very potent topical steroids are usually required to reduce the inflammation and stop the itching. Antihistamines do not help. Intralesional steroids are effective, and occlusion with coal tar bandages is often successful.

Asteatotic eczema

Introduction

This is also known as xerosis, winter itch, and eczema craquelé, and is a disease of the elderly characterized by dry cracked skin that may have been subjected to excessive bathing and scrubbing.

Clinical features

The skin becomes degreased by washing, and chapped (= dried and cracked) by the cold. The legs, particularly the shins, are affected, and sometimes the trunk and arms.

Treatment

Topical steroids diluted in white soft paraffin reduce itching and heal the skin. 'Greasing' agents such as emulsifying ointment are used as soap substitutes. Healing is usually rapid and continual use of 'greasing' agents prevents recurrence.

Hypostatic eczema

Introduction

This eczema occurs on the inner aspect of the shin, just above the medial malleolus, following hypostasis, i.e. poor tissue perfusion due to high venous pressure, that may result from circulatory problems, e.g. postphlebitic syndrome, or incompetent valves in the venous system of the legs.

Clinical features

Middle-aged and elderly women are particularly affected. Initially there is itching followed by a dry scaly area, which may become erythematous (Figure 17) and purpuric. There may be an accumulation of thick greasy scales, but usually the skin tends to become thinner, shiny, hyperpigmented and friable.

Problems

Ulceration, secondary infection, and generally poor healing are all-too-common problems. Additionally, allergic contact and irritant eczemas can more easily develop in these areas of thin and broken skin, and may then become disseminated. Prolonged severe hypostatic eczema itself may similarly become generalized by autosensitization; this is a process by which any eczema – endogenous or exogenous – can disseminate, in some patients a delayed type response to their own epidermal antigens being demonstrated. Some autosensitization occurs in characteristic patterns, for example, hypostatic eczema spreading to the arms, and nickel sensitivity to the eyes; sometimes it may be difficult to differentiate between autosensitization of endogenous eczema and superimposition of allergic contact eczema.

Management

The cause of the hypostatsis must be determined and treated if possible and this may involve venography. Postural drainage to counteract the high venous pressure is helpful. At night the foot of the bed should be raised 22–23cm (9 inches). Patients should be encouraged to lie on the bed for an hour in the afternoon. Standing and sitting with the legs down are bad for the condition, but exercise – since the muscle pump encourages venous drainage – is good. If patients do sit they should elevate their legs, the higher the better. If ulceration develops this should be treated by cleaning the ulcer with equal parts eusol and paraffin, and then dressed with a non-adhesive dressing. A firm supportive bandage from the toes to the knee should be worn. Patients often find a cotton bandage impregnated with zinc oxide next to the skin under an Elastoplast bandage very helpful. These bandages need only be changed weekly.

Overall treatment may be long and difficult, and a sympathetic and encouraging approach from a well-coordinated medical team is as important as a cooperative and well-motivated patient.

7

PSORIASIS

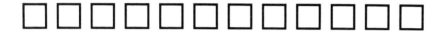

INTRODUCTION

Psoriasis is a common disorder, and it has been estimated to affect 2% of the population in the United Kingdom. The exact cause of psoriasis is unknown but there are strong suggestions that genetic factors play an important role. However, other factors are undoubtedly necessary in the clinical expression of the disease. Only one third of patients with psoriasis have a family history of the complaint in a first degree relative. It would appear that the predisposition for the disease is inherited and other factors may precipitate the disorder. The known triggers for psoriasis include streptococcal infections, trauma to the skin, mental stress, and certain drugs, e.g. lithium salts and chloroquin. However, these trigger factors are only found in a minority of patients.

Psoriasis is characterized by proliferation of the epidermal cells and a maturation defect of these cells, with the result that an abnormal keratin layer forms. There is now some evidence that this proliferation of cells is mediated by immunological mechanisms, most probably mediated via the T-lymphocytes.

CLINICAL FEATURES

Psoriasis affects the sexes equally. It may appear for the first time at any age, but is very rare before the age of 5, and uncommon before the age of 15. The disorder most commonly presents in young adult life and the incidence of first presentation gradually falls from middle age. However, the disorder may appear for the first time in the eighth and ninth decades.

The clinical features of psoriasis may vary depending on the site of involvement, e.g. palms and soles, and flexural regions may have a different appearance to the lesions at other sites. The commoner sites of involvement are the extensor surfaces of the knees and elbows, followed by the scalp and sacral region, but any part of the skin may be affected (Figure 18). The typical lesion of psoriasis is a well-demarcated red, raised patch with white scales (Figure 19). The scales are loosely bound and gentle scratching with a wooden spatula shows flaking of the lesion and increases the whiteness of the lesion. If all the scales are removed with the spatula capillary bleeding points are seen. The extent of involvement in psoriasis varies considerably, from a few patches to total involvement of the skin surface.

Scalp

Psoriasis may affect the scalp with or without lesions elsewhere. In the scalp the involvement may vary from a solitary patch to the whole of the scalp. The lesions usually stop at the hairline. Examination shows well-demarcated patches with an irregularly 'lumpy' surface, the excess and abnormal keratin adhering to the hair and not being as easily shed as the scales elsewhere.

Palms and soles

At these sites psoriasis may present with discrete patches or be confluent. When the lesions are patchy they present as firm hyperkeratotic yellowish brown areas with adherent scale, unlike the lesions elsewhere. If the involvement is confluent, the palms and soles are red with some scaling, and there is a sharp line of demarcation between the involved and non-involved skin at the sides of the palms and soles. Occasionally psoriasis only affects the palms and soles with no lesions elsewhere and the diagnosis can be difficult.

Nails

The nails are affected in approximately 50% of patients with psoriasis. The commonest feature is small pits. The other features include onycholysis (separation of the nail plate from the nail bed), subungual hyperkeratosis and dystrophy (breaking of nail). Occasionally involvement of the nails occurs without skin lesions.

Flexural psoriasis

When psoriasis affects the groins, perianal skin and axillae, it appears as well-demarcated red areas with a shiny surface. The white dry scales are not present because of the moisture of these areas. Occasionally painful fissures may occur, particularly in the posterior natal cleft. As with psoriasis localized to other areas, the disorder may be localized to the intertriginous areas, and give rise to difficulty in diagnosis.

Guttate psoriasis

This is a term used to denote the sudden appearance of numerous small lesions of psoriasis, usually on the trunk (Figure 20). Subsequently similar lesions may appear on the limbs. The lesions are red but with minimal scaling, but this is increased on excoriation. The distinctive feature of guttate psoriasis is that in the majority of patients the disorder is self-limiting, the lesions disappearing within 3 months of onset. Guttate psoriasis is most common in children and young adults, and one of the known triggers is a streptococcal infection.

Erythrodermic psoriasis

This is the term used when psoriasis involves the whole of the skin surface. The patient presents with erythema and scaling. However the scaling is different to that seen in plaques of psoriasis, and is not so thick and does not always have a white appearance on excoriation. This may be due to the fact that erythrodermic psoriasis is the most active form of the disease, and less keratin is produced than in chronic plaque psoriasis. Patients with erythrodermic psoriasis lose a great deal of heat and often are seen to be shivering in order to maintain their body temperature. These patients are at risk from hypothermia.

Pustular psoriasis

There are two types of pustular psoriasis.

One is the localized form seen on the palms and soles, where the condition presents as red, scaly patches with small pustules (Figure 21). These lesions are sterile. Localized pustular psoriasis is usually but not always symmetrical. The condition tends to be persistent and has been termed 'persistent eruption of the palms and soles'.

The other form of pustular psoriasis is the generalized one. In this condition sheets of small pustules appear in extensive psoriatic lesions on the trunk and limbs. The patients usually have a fever and constitutional upset. This form of psoriasis is very rare.

Koebner phenomenon

This is the term applied to psoriasis appearing at the sites of trauma. It is seen after falls, cuts, thermal burns and severe sunburn.

Arthropathy

Five per cent of patients with psoriasis develop an arthropathy. It is similar in its distribution to rheumatoid arthritis except that the terminal interphalangeal joint is involved in psoriasis. The disorder can also be distinguished from rheumatoid arthritis by the fact that the rheumatoid factor is absent.

As in rheumatoid arthritis psoriatic involvement of the joints may be mild and self-limiting, or there may be severe involvement leading to permanent damage and deformity of the joints. The condition may also affect one or only a few joints, or there may be extensive involvement. Psoriatic arthropathy may occur without skin lesions.

Prognosis

The course of psoriasis is variable. In some individuals the disease is limited to a few persistent patches on the elbows or knees, whilst in others the disease becomes extensive. It has been estimated that 40% of patients can expect spontaneous remissions. The factors which control the extent and persistence of the lesions are not known.

PROBLEMS

Typical psoriatic lesions do not usually present a problem in diagnosis. However, when the disease is localized to certain sites the diagnosis may be difficult. If the scalp alone is involved the condition has to be distinguished from seborrhoeic eczema. The latter tends to have flatter lesions and not heaped keratotic plaques.

Acute guttate psoriasis has to be distinguished from pityriasis rosea and secondary syphilis. In pityriasis rosea, there may be a herald patch and centripetal scaling of the oval lesions. Secondary syphilis may be associated with lesions on the palms and soles and ulcers in the mouth.

Psoriasis involving only the palms and soles has to be distinguished from chronic eczema. The line of demarcation between the affected and non-affected skin is more marked in psoriasis. If the lesions are not confluent but present as small plaques, the condition has to be distinguished from lichen planus at these sites.

Nail involvement in psoriasis has to be distinguished from a fungal infection. Pits are not usually seen in fungal infections, but onycholysis, subungual hyperkeratosis and dystrophy may occur in both conditions. Specimens must be taken for mycology if there is doubt as to the diagnosis.

Flexural or intertriginous psoriasis may be confused with intertriginous eczema, fungal infections and erythrasma. If only the intertriginous areas are involved it may be impossible to distinguish between eczema and psoriasis. Ringworm fungal infections tend to have a raised scaly edge. Erythrasma often has a reddish brown colour as opposed to bright red, and the diagnosis can be made by microscopy of skin scrapings which will show the organisms causing erythrasma.

Pustular psoriasis on the palms and soles has to be distinguished from secondarily infected eczema or fungal infections. If there is doubt, specimens should be taken for mycology and bacteriology. Generalized pustular psoriasis has to be differentiated from widespread impetigo, pemphigus, and a rare condition called subcorneal pustular dermatosis.

Erythroderma due to eczema has the same appearance as that due to psoriasis, and the preceding history may give the exact diagnosis. The Sezary syndrome and mycosis fungoides, which are skin reticuloses, may also give rise to erythroderma.

ASSESSMENT AND INVESTIGATIONS

No investigations are usually required as the diagnosis can be made on the clinical features. However, if there is doubt a biopsy will be necessary. Skin scrapings should be taken for mycological examination if there is doubt as to whether the disorder is a fungal infection. In acute guttate psoriasis the VDRL may be necessary if there is a possibility of the rash being a secondary syphilitic eruption. If there is joint involvement, serological tests for the rheumatoid factor and uric acid level should be carried out.

MANAGEMENT

General

It is important to explain the nature of the condition to the patient and stress the non-contagious aspect of the disorder. Patients should be told that at present no permanent cure exists, but that the condition can always be cleared and controlled if necessary, and that a large proportion will achieve a spontaneous remission.

If psoriasis is active, then whatever treatment is given the condition is likely to relapse when treatment is discontinued, whereas if the disorder is not active, a long remission may be obtained with the same treatment. The activity of psoriasis can be judged by a number of clinical features. If the condition is extensive or new lesions are developing then the disease is active, whereas if the lesions are not increasing in size and no new ones are appearing, this suggests low activity. Plaques which show clearing from the centre often imply spontaneous resolution of these lesions.

Topical steroids

These are the most commonly prescribed drugs for psoriasis. As a general rule weak topical steroids are ineffective in clearing psoriasis and the stronger the steroid the greater its antipsoriatic effect. Short courses (2 weeks) of potent topical steroids are justified in the treatment of psoriasis, but they should not be used on the face or intertriginous areas. If the psoriasis recurs within a few weeks, this implies active disease and potent topical steroids should not be used again. As a general rule, potent topical steroids should not be used for longer than 2-week periods, every 2 months. If they are used on a continuous basis tachyphylaxis may occur, i.e. more topical steroid is required to achieve the same clinical result.

Moderate-strength topical steroids are sometimes used for longer periods, if they are capable of suppressing or partially suppressing the disorder, but close supervision is required.

The advantage of topical steroids is that, compared to other topical preparations, they are pleasant to use. The disadvantage of topical steroids is that if they are used for any length of time there is a risk of collagen atrophy to the skin. The stronger the steroid, the more likely are side-effects to occur. Clinically collagen atrophy presents as spontaneous bruising, telangiectasia and striae and the skin looks thin.

As a general rule, topical steroids in psoriasis should be used in an ointment rather than a cream or lotion base, except for the intertriginous areas.

Coal tar preparations

These are not used very frequently today. Crude coal tar is effective in the treatment of psoriasis but the purified tar preparations are not so effective. However, crude coal tar preparations are unpleasant to use as they are messy and have a strong smell of tar. If coal tar is to be used, it is usually employed at an initial strength of 5% and is made up into an ointment, e.g. white soft paraffin, or paste as a base. To clear psoriasis with coal tar preparations usually takes approximately 4 weeks; and patients usually have to be admitted to hospital for extensive disease. It is important that the lesions when treated are covered by tube gauze dressings to protect the clothes and bedding.

Liquid coal tar is still used for bathing in patients with psoriasis. It is either added to the bath water (approximately 30ml) or else 15% liquid coal tar in emulsifying ointment B.P. can be applied to the skin prior to bathing.

Dithranol

Structurally this is similar to tars. Dithranol is a highly effective agent in clearing psoriasis. It has two main drawbacks, however.

Firstly it will stain the surrounding skin, clothes, and bed linen a purple colour, and this staining is permanent on clothes and linen. The staining lasts about 2 weeks on the skin after discontinuing the treatment. The second disadvantage is that dithranol is an irritant to the skin surrounding the psoriatic lesions. This irritation presents as erythema and a burning sensation; if it is severe there may be blister formation and soreness. In an attempt to limit these side-effects, dithranol is applied in a paste to stop the spread to the surrounding skin. Lassar's paste (which contains 2% salicylic acid) is a suitable medium. It is usual to start at a concentration of 0.1% dithranol and gradually increase the strength to 0.5% depending on the clinical response and side-effects. More recently, 2% dithranol has been used, applied for only 1 hour per day. The advantage of using a high concentration for a short duration is that the treatment can be given on an outpatient basis. If the dithranol is applied for 24 hours it will have to be covered with tube gauze dressings to protect the clothes and linen.

Dithranol usually takes 3–4 weeks to clear psoriasis. It should not be used on the face, genitalia or intertriginous areas.

Ultraviolet light

It has long been known that sunlight tends to have a beneficial effect on psoriasis. As a rule the stronger the sun, the better the effect. UVB (middle-wave ultraviolet light) can be used as the sole treatment. However, high intensity lamps are required and it takes approximately 6 weeks to clear the lesions. The treatment is usually carried out three times per week. Once the psoriasis is cleared, weekly maintenance treatment may keep the patient clear of lesions.

PUVA (photochemotherapy)

PUVA is derived from P for psoralens and UVA (long-wave ultraviolet light). Psoralens are drugs which act as photosensitizers, and have a number of biological effects in the presence of ultraviolet. UVA is employed as there is no 'sunburn' effect, as happens with UVB. PUVA is a highly effective treatment in clearing psoriasis. The treatment is usually carried out three times a week, and it takes 4–5 weeks to clear psoriasis. Maintenance treatment either weekly or every 2 weeks can be given to stop a recurrence. The disadvantage of PUVA is that it is time-consuming for the patient to attend the hospital three times a week. The possible long-term side-effect of continuous PUVA is the possible carcinogenic effects of the UVA. However, after 8 years' experience of PUVA there has been no epidemic of skin malignancy in patients who have had long-term PUVA.

Retinoids

The drug etretinate has been used in psoriasis for the past 2–3 years. However, it is not effective in clearing the disease in more than 50% of patients. Its side-effects include dry lips and mild facial scaling. The long-term side-effects include possible elevation of the blood lipids. It is teratogenic and therefore should be used with caution in women of childbearing age.

Cytotoxic drugs

These are not used so frequently since the advent of PUVA. The most effective and safest drug for psoriasis is methotrexate. It should be given as a once-weekly dose; there is a risk of hepatic fibrosis when it is used long term.

Treatment for special sites

Scalp

Psoriasis of the scalp is difficult to treat. It is difficult to apply topical preparations because of the hair, and ultraviolet light and

PUVA are not effective. Topical preparations that are helpful have to be used in a lotion base or, if ointment or cream, have to be applied at night and be washed out the following morning. There are several topical corticosteroid preparations but they do not always appear to be effective and as a rule should not be used continuously. Simple keratolytics are often helpful because they decrease the scaling, which is often the main cause of embarrassment to the patient. Salicylic acid 5% and sulphur 5% in aqueous cream B.P. applied two or three times a week at night is often all that is necessary. A more effective but somewhat unpleasant preparation is : solution coal tar 10%, salicylic acid 5%, sulphur 5%, coconut oil 40% and emulsifying ointment 40%. This preparation should also only be used at night and washed out the next morning; the frequency of use will depend on the severity of the condition.

Flexural intertriginous psoriasis

The only topical treatment that should be used is short courses of moderate or strong topical steroids in a cream base. Fortunately they are usually effective. Continuous treatment should be avoided if possible.

Psoriatic arthropathy

The treatment for this is the same as for rheumatoid arthritis. In the mild forms salicylates and other non-steroidal anti-inflammatory drugs may be used. In severe cases gold or immunosuppressive drugs may help. Systemic steroids should be avoided because, when the dose is reduced, there may be a flare-up of the skin lesions.

Referral to specialist

If the psoriasis is not extensive and the nature of the condition is accepted by the patient, then referral to a specialist is unnecessary.

However, some patients do not accept the fact there are some diseases in the 1980s that cannot be cured by medical science, and a second opinion may be necessary to enlighten them. If psoriasis is severe and incapacitating then referral will be necessary.

8

LICHEN PLANUS

☐ ☐ ☐ ☐ ☐ ☐ ☐ ☐ ☐ ☐ ☐ ☐

INTRODUCTION

Lichen planus is a distinct clinical entity of unknown aetiology. Infective agents, particularly viruses and mycoplasma, have been implicated as the cause of lichen planus, but there is no evidence that this is so. It is not uncommon, accounting for 1% of new patients in dermatological clinics in the UK.

CLINICAL FEATURES

Lichen planus may occur at any age but is uncommon in childhood and the elderly. The typical lesion is a violaceous, flat-topped, shiny papule varying in size from 2 to 5mm. White streaks may be seen on the surface; these are known as 'Wickham's striae'. The commonest sites of involvement are the wrists and flexor aspect of the forearms (Figure 22), lumbar region and ankles, but any part of the skin and mucous membranes may be affected. Lichen planus often occurs at the site of trauma giving a linear configuration to the lesion. (This is the so-called Koebner phenomenon.) Lichen planus may or may not be associated with pruritus. Depending on the anatomical site the lesions of lichen planus may be modified, giving different lesions.

Palms and soles

When lichen planus involves these areas the lesions present as hyperkeratotic, yellow brown papules which frequently merge to form plaques.

Legs

On the lower legs lichen planus presents as raised violaceous scaly plaques. This is sometimes known as hypertrophic lichen planus.

Scalp

At this site lichen planus presents with violaceous plaques; when these resolve they may leave atrophic skin with subsequent hair loss.

Mucous membranes

The mouth is a common site of involvement and lesions may occur without involvement elsewhere. The commonest site to be affected in the oral cavity is the buccal mucosa and the lesions present as white papules or streaks with a smooth surface. The gums may also be involved and at this site the disease presents as erythematous shiny areas, and not infrequently erosions occur (erosive lichen planus). Superficial erosions and ulcers may also appear on the buccal mucosa. Erosive lichen planus is often a very painful disorder, and the patients have difficulty eating.

The vulva and vagina may also be affected and the lesions are similar to those seen in the oral cavity and may also break down to present as ulcers and erosions. Erosive lichen planus of the vulva will give rise to dyspareunia. On the glans penis the characteristic lesions are annular, white, raised lesions.

Nails

Involvement of the nails is rare. When it occurs there is longitudinal ridging; if this is severe the nail is destroyed, with pterygium formation, i.e. the skin from the posterior nail fold growing forward on the nail bed with loss of the nail plate.

Bullae

Occasionally the lichen planus lesions on the skin may give rise to bullae.

Follicular

A rare form of presentation is when lichen planus is confined to the hair follicles.

DURATION

In the majority of patients lichen planus is a self-limiting disorder resolving within a year of onset. Sometimes, however, the disorder is persistent, lasting for years, and this is often the case when it affects the mucous membranes. A small proportion of patients have a second bout of lichen planus.

PROBLEMS

Pruritus is a common feature. There may be difficulty in eating when there is erosive lichen planus of the mouth and dyspareunia when there is involvement of the vulva. Squamous cell carcinoma is a rare complication of longstanding lesions in the mouth.

The papular variety of lichen planus must be distinguished from guttate psoriasis, secondary syphilis and some forms of eczema in which the lesions tend to be papular. A drug eruption may sometimes be lichenoid. The drugs which usually give rise to this eruption are isoniazid, mepacrine and gold.

Hypertrophic lichen planus is most likely to be confused with localized lichenified eczema (lichen simplex). The papular and linear mucous membrane lesions have to be distinguished from *Candida* infection and leukoplakia. When the mucosal lesions ulcerate, the differential diagnosis includes pemphigus, benign mucous membrane pemphigoid, infective causes of gingivitis, recurrent aphthous ulcers and possibly Behçet's disease. In addition the vulval lesions have to be distinguished from recurrent herpes simplex infection.

ASSESSMENT AND INVESTIGATION

The diagnosis can usually be made on clinical examination. If there is doubt a biopsy should be performed. Tests may also be necessary to exclude syphilis, pemphigus, mucous membrane pemphigoid and *Candida* infections.

MANAGEMENT

Once the diagnosis has been established and the disorder is not giving rise to symptoms, no treatment is necessary. Reassurance should be given as to the benign and non-infective nature of the disease.

Topical

If there is severe irritation or patients are concerned about the appearance of the rash, strong or very strong topical steroids should be used for 2 or 3 weeks and they may be effective in clearing the rash. These preparations should not be used indefinitely. Weaker topical steroids may be effective in controlling the irritation but will probably not clear the rash.

Betamethasone 17-valerate (Betnovate) mouth pellets (obtained from Glaxo) are often effective in healing the oral lesions. Topical steroids should be used for vulval lesions.

Intralesional injections of triamcinolone may clear hypertrophic lichen planus.

Systemic treatment

Steroids are effective in clearing lichen planus. Prednisone 20mg daily given for 2 weeks is usually sufficient. However, if the disease is active the condition will recur. Maintenance treatment with steroids is probably not justified.

PUVA (psoralens plus UVA) is also effective in clearing lichen planus and should be considered in widespread disease. Maintenance treatment will be necessary if the disease is active.

The retinoid, etretinate, has been reported to be helpful in erosive lichen planus.

Oral antihistamines have a small part to play in controlling pruritus.

Referral to specialist

This is necessary if there is doubt about the diagnosis or for assessment of treatment if the disorder is extensive and difficult to control with courses of topical and systemic steroids.

Long-term care

This should generally not be necessary, as in the majority of patients the disease will go into remission. Long-term care may be necessary in mucous membrane lesions and this probably would be supervised by a specialist.

9

PITYRIASIS ROSEA

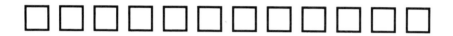

INTRODUCTION

This is a common dermatosis of unknown aetiology, although a virus is suspected; it is certainly very uncommon for patients to have a second attack – suggesting that immunity is gained against a virus. The term pityriasis is derived from the Greek word for 'branlike'. The disorder occurs more commonly in temperate climes (usually in the spring or autumn) and affects mainly young adults.

CLINICAL FEATURES

The eruption often begins with a solitary 'herald patch', which is a pink, slightly indurated, scaly, oval or annular lesion. The patch is larger than subsequent lesions and usually occurs on the trunk. The patient may complain of a mild sore throat and malaise at this stage. Within 1–2 weeks the eruption proper appears, mostly on the trunk, occasionally extending to the neck and upper parts of the limbs, and rarely affecting the face, hands and feet. The lesions are oval and pink with centripetal scaling and tend to lie with their long axes in the line of cleavage of the skin, most obvious around the side of the chest wall. Occasionally the lesions tend to be

73

papular. The condition rarely causes any problems apart from minimal irritation, and the rash clears within 2–3 months.

PROBLEMS

The initial 'herald patch' may be confused with a tinea infection but skin scrapings and development of the full rash will clarify the picture. In most cases diagnosis is easy, but occasionally there are only a few lesions or the rash is not typical and the condition may have to be distinguished from a seborrhoeic eczema, or a guttate psoriasis, or a drug eruption. The important differential diagnosis always to bear in mind is secondary syphilis, so a careful history is essential, and the presence of other secondary syphilis lesions, particularly papules on the palms and soles, all help to distinguish the condition, although serological tests should be carried out if there is any doubt.

TREATMENT

The patient is reassured as to the benign and self-limiting nature of the condition and usually no active treatment is required. If necessary, the lesions and any irritation can be suppressed with moderate-strength topical steroids, and oral antihistamines may be of help in some cases.

10

ACNE

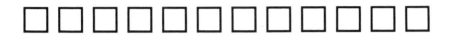

INTRODUCTION

Acne is a common disease of the sebaceous glands and ducts, affecting mainly the face, trunk and shoulders, and occurring mostly in adolescents, but in some cases persisting into late middle age. Rarely it occurs in the first 2 years of life, tending to fade by the age of 5.

Several processes play a part in the development of acne.

(1) Alteration of sebaceous duct lining cells causes obstruction of the ducts.

(2) Abnormal sebum production leads to altered quality or increased amounts which either blocks the ducts or renders the sebum more inflammatory.

(3) Bacterial colonization with *Propionibacterium acnes* modifies the sebum or releases mediators of inflammation.

Blocking of the duct leads to comedone formation; when the orifice of the duct is visible the horny plug forms an open comedone or 'blackhead' and if the orifice is closed, a white papule or closed comedone is formed. The blocked duct causes distension of the sebaceous gland, thus exciting a foreign body reaction, with further inflammation sometimes being caused by rupture of the gland into the dermis.

The sex hormones have a profound effect on acne. Induction and exacerbation of acne may be associated with:

(1) presence of excess androgens,

(2) relative excess due to diminished oestrogen,

(3) low sex hormone binding globulin leading to high free plasma testosterone or

(4) increased peripheral uptake of androgen.

Taking a high oestrogen content contraceptive pill can improve acne, whereas pills containing the newer synthetic progesterones such as norgestrel have an antioestrogenic activity which may exacerbate acne.

In addition to hormonal disturbance leading to acne, a defect in cell-mediated immunity has been reported in cases of severe acne, when additional damage due to deposition of immune complexes may occur.

CLINICAL FEATURES

Acne lesions occur mostly on face, shoulders and trunk. Chin and forehead are often the first sites to be affected. Premenstrual flares are commonly confined to the chin, and in older women the 'beard' area is predominantly involved. In the severe and disfiguring acne conglobata the lesions extend to upper arms, buttocks and thighs. The distribution of lesions in acne, due to exogenous factors, varies according to the exact cause.

The comedone is the initial lesion. Surrounding inflammation causes erythematous papules and pustules, and in severe cases cysts and nodules which are persistent. There may be associated seborrhoea manifest as greasy skin and hair. Postinflammatory hyperpigmentation may occur. Depressed pitted scars or keloids may form.

Rarely, severe cystic acne in teenage boys may be accompanied by fever and joint pains, and erythema nodosum, with leukocytosis and raised erythrocyte sedimentation rate.

Acne conglobata, the severe disfiguring form of acne, may arise in pre-existing acne or in patients whose disease has remitted, and the condition tends to persist often beyond the age of 50. There is often a strong family history. The severe inflammatory response leads to abscess formation and discharging interconnecting sinuses. Febrile episodes may occur. Cysts and nodules are numerous and may ulcerate and become necrotic. Scarring is severe, often with keloid formation. There may be associated hidradenitis suppruativa of apocrine glands in axillae, groins and breast.

PROBLEMS

Management of cosmetically embarrassed patients presents great difficulty. It is unfair to evade the problems of treatment and difficulty of 'cure', by suggesting that the condition is only adolescent, physiological, and self-limiting, when often the activity of the disease can cause great problems and persist much longer. The doctor must strive for exacting treatments and give support and encouragement in his consultations.

Differential diagnosis may be a problem with similar rashes being caused by rosacea and perioral dermatitis, but localization and absence of comedones usually delineate the latter conditions. Pustular pseudofolliculitis barbae and follicular seborrhoeic eczema may cause confusion. Exogenous acne is usually differentiated by localization and predominance of comedones.

ASSESSMENT AND INVESTIGATION

Infantile acne may be the presenting symptom of a virilizing syndrome such as congenital adrenal hyperplasia; physical examination and biochemical study should therefore be carried out.

Women with severe and resistant acne, facial hirsutism and infrequent menstruation should be investigated for polycystic ovaries; if there is amenorrhoea and virilization of external genitalia, investigations should be made for androgen-secreting tumours. The above are uncommon conditions, and in most cases of acne there is no difficulty with diagnosis and no investigation is required.

MANAGEMENT

Keratolytics are useful in treating the superficial pustules and comedones of mild acne. After washing with antiseptic soap, nightly applications of preparations such as salicylic acid (1–3%), benzoyl peroxide (5–10%) and resorcinol (1–3%) are used to cause slight erythema and peeling.

Ultraviolet light can also help by virtue of its peeling effect, but perhaps more so by its masking effect through tanning.

Retinoic acid preparations cause irritation and peeling, and also alteration of sebaceous duct keratinization, but severe irritant reactions and hyperpigmentation may occur.

Topical clindamycin as 1 or 1.5% lotion is now commonly used and is sometimes very helpful. Systemic absorption is low. Oral clindamycin (150mg daily) is occasionally given but higher doses should not be used because of the risk of enterocolitis.

The sytemic antibiotics commonly used in acne therapy are tetracyclines (250mg b.d.), erythromycin (250mg b.d.) minocycline (50mg b.d.) and co-trimoxazole (Septrin, 1 b.d.) There is little response within 1 month's treatment and effectiveness is difficult to assess before 3 months, after which time reduction to maintenance dosage should be considered. In difficult cases treatment may need to be continued for many years.

Dapsone in high doses (100–300mg daily) and corticosteroids in moderate doses are occasionally used in severe resistant cystic acne.

Antiandrogen treatment is becoming more widely used in acne

therapy for women because of an undoubted high success rate and also reduced recurrence rate after terminating treatment. The drug used is cyproterone acetate. The most effective regimen is to take cyproterone acetate 50 mg daily from the fifth to the fourteenth day of the menstrual cycle, and ethinyl oestradiol 50 μg from the fifth to the twenty-sixth day of the cycle. Oestrogens have to be taken to regulate the menstrual cycle and provide contraception. A small dose of cyproterone acetate 2 mg daily combined with ethinyl oestradiol 50 μg daily from the fifth to the twenty-sixth days of the cycle (as found in the contraceptive pill, Diane) has also been used, but is not as effective as the higher dose of cyproterone acetate. However, in patients with mild acne, or a past history of severe acne, Diane should be considered as a suitable oral contraceptive. It is also important to bear in mind that contraceptive pills containing progesterones with androgenic properties (e.g. norgestrel) may aggravate or precipitate acne in susceptible individuals.

Cyproterone acetate reduces the cutaneous effects of androgens as well as reducing testosterone levels by inhibiting gonadotrophins. The oestrogen also reduces ovarian production of androgens and raises sex hormone binding globulin, thus lowering plasma free testosterone. It is important to remember, however, that the oestrogen component also introduces the possibility of extra side-effects and the same criteria as used for selection of patients for use of the contraceptive pill must be applied to selection of those for this regime.

Improvement in acne with cyproterone acetate therapy is generally seen within 30 days and clearing in 80 days. To date, treatment tends to have been reserved for severe cases of female acne, but it may well become a standard treatment in less severe cases. The drug is also used in idiopathic hirsutism and androgenic diffuse alopecia in women.

13-*cis*-Retinoic acid (isotretinoin) is a recently introduced oral retinoid which suppresses sebum production and reduces keratinization of the hair follicle. It has revolutionized the treatment of severe cystic acne. It is given daily (0.5–1 mg/kg body weight) for 4 months, and usually eliminates cyst formation, with effects lasting for 6–12 months after stopping treatment. Like all oral retinoids, it is a teratogenic drug with persistence of effects for 1 month after termination of treatment, so strict contraceptive precautions must be observed in women patients. Other problems that may be encountered are dryness of the lips and elevation of serum lipids.

Large persistent acne cysts can be treated by syringe or Dermo-jet injection of steroids which reduce inflammatory reaction, improve resolution and reduce scarring. Post-acne scarring can be helped in some cases by dermabrasion, and occasionally by injection of collagen preparations, but the latter are not permanent.

11

ROSACEA

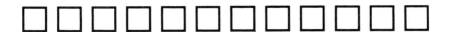

INTRODUCTION

Rosacea is a distinct clinical entity, the cause of which is unknown. The principle changes occur in the blood vessels and sebaceous glands on the face. There is dilatation of the superficial blood vessels and new vessel formation. The sebaceous glands are hypertrophied and surrounded by inflammatory changes, and granuloma formation may occur.

CLINICAL FEATURES

Rosacea is most commonly seen in middle-aged adults, but may occur in young adults and the elderly. It is invariably confined to the face. The first sign is often flushing of the face due to the usual stimuli such as anxiety, alcohol and spicy food. The flushing eventually tends to be persistent, giving persistent erythema. Other features of the disorder then appear – telangiectasia, red papules and pustules (Figure 23). The lesions may be widespread and involve the whole face or they may occur only on the forehead, cheeks, nose or chin. Very occasionally papules and pustules may occur without background erythema. Rosacea is usually symmetrical.

A variant of rosacea is rhinophyma. It is most commonly seen in men and there may be no features of rosacea elsewhere. Rhinophyma is thickening of the skin on the nose and often presents as an irregular lobulated mass. It is due to hyperplasia of the connective tissue and sebaceous glands.

In addition to the skin, the eye may be affected in rosacea. There may be blepharitis, conjunctivitis and occasionally keratitis. In the latter there is corneal vascularization. Eye involvement is present in nearly half the patients.

Rosacea tends to be a persistent disorder and may last for many years, although eventually spontaneous remission will occur in a large proportion of patients. Rhinophyma is persistent and does not tend to involute.

PROBLEMS

Rosacea has to be distinguished from acne, in which there is usually no background erythema and comedones may be seen. Bacterial folliculitis which presents as papules and pustules does not usually have background erythema. Systemic lupus erythematosus characteristically affects the nose and cheeks and there are no papules or pustules. Seborrhoeic and contact eczema may present with erythema but there is usually scaling. Carcinoid syndrome may present as flushing attacks and eventually persistent erythema. Possibly one of the most common conditions to mimic rosacea is seen after the use of potent topical steroids on the face. There is erythema and telangiectasia, and papules and pustules may be present particularly around the mouth – so-called circumoral dermatitis.

ASSESSMENT AND INVESTIGATION

The diagnosis can usually be made on clinical grounds. If there is doubt about the diagnosis, investigation may be necessary to exclude some of the conditions mentioned above.

MANAGEMENT

The majority of patients with rosacea respond to oral tetracycline. The initial dose is 250mg b.d. and should be given for 6 weeks. If there is considerable improvement or clearing after this time, the dose should be reduced to 250mg daily for a further 6 weeks. If tetracycline is discontinued, two thirds of patients will relapse within 6 months. Thus the majority of patients do need permanent treatment; often 250mg daily or on alternate days is sufficient to suppress the disorder. If patients have had no lesions for 3 months while taking a maintenance dose, they should be instructed to discontinue treatment to see if permanent spontaneous resolution has occurred.

A small proportion of patients do not clear with tetracycline, and the other drug which is effective is metronidazole. The dose is 200mg b.d., and the regimen is similar to that with tetracycline. Recently there have been reports of successful treatment with topical 1% metronidazole in a cream base.

Tetracycline also appears to clear the ocular lesions of rosacea but has little or no effect on rhinophyma, which has to be treated by surgical shaving usually carried out by a plastic surgeon.

Referral to specialist

This is not necessary if the diagnosis is made and the condition responds to tetracycline. Referrals are only necessary if the clinical diagnosis is in doubt or there is failure to respond to treatment.

Long-term care

Patients will have to be seen if only for repeat prescriptions of tetracycline. Patients should be told to discontinue treatment if clear for 3 months. If relapse does occur they should start treatment again.

12

URTICARIA

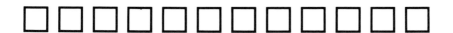

INTRODUCTION

This is localized oedema of the skin or mucous membranes of the upper respiratory tract due to acute vasodilatation and increased permeability of capillaries following release of various chemical mediators such as histamine from degranulated mast cells .

The condition is often referred to as 'hives' or 'nettle rash', and can be precipitated by various factors, most commonly drugs, especially penicillins and salicylates, some foods, particularly shellfish, and also by heat, cold, sunlight, insect bites, and trauma (as exhibited by dermographism). Psychological stress and physical debilitating illness are probably aggravating rather than causative factors. Needless to say, most cases of urticaria, especially the chronic type, are of unknown cause.

CLINICAL FEATURES

The initial lesion is an itchy erythematous patch which subsequently becomes raised and then white at the centre due to pressure of oedema. The size of the patch may vary from a few millimetres to a large confluent area with irregular outline – this is mostly on the trunk and limbs, whereas on the hands and feet the lesions are limited, being tense, red and swollen. Involvement of the face causes swelling around the eyes and/or lips, sometimes known as angioneurotic oedema, when it may be associated with swelling of tongue, pharynx and larynx. Bronchospasm, gut colic, joint effusions and even anaphylactic shock may occur in association with urticaria.

The condition runs an extremely variable course, the acute lesions lasting from as little as a few minutes to several days, with chronic lesions tending to disperse and recur in varying sites in an entirely unpredictable manner. Chronic urticaria may last for months or years.

PROBLEMS

The main difficulties are concerned with (1) determining the precipitating cause and (2) managing chronic urticaria. A careful history is important, particularly regarding drug and food intake. If a drug is suspected it should be stopped and avoided in the future. Skin tests are unhelpful and oral provocation tests with drugs and foods – including food additives, dyes and preservatives – are notoriously difficult to evaluate, as are elimination diets, mainly because the condition runs such a variable course. Occasionally it is established that the urticaria is caused or aggravated by specific physical factors such as heat and cold, and these factors can then be avoided.

The treatment of chronic or recurring urticaria is difficult and often antihistamines need to be given in high dosage – fortunately some of the more recently produced antihistamines such as astemizole and terfenadine have a much reduced sedative side-effect. Additionally, time must be spent with the patient for explanation and advice about the condition as it is often a disheartening problem which may be compounded by anxiety.

MANAGEMENT

Because the epidermis is intact in urticaria, current topical drugs are ineffective. Oral antihistamines are the mainstay of treatment, the dosage being gradually increased until the urticaria is controlled or side-effects become unacceptable, though fortunately this limitation is receding with availability of the newer drugs, as mentioned above. The serotonin antagonist, cyproheptadine, and hydroxyzine are drugs occasionally used when antihistamines fail.

In severe or acute urticaria the antihistamines can be given by intramuscular or intravenous injection, often in conjunction with steroids, especially if there is involvement of tongue or larynx, or if there is associated anaphylactic shock. Subcutaneous adrenaline is also useful in these circumstances. Hopefully, use of these drugs will obviate the need for tracheotomy.

Psychotropic drugs are occasionally helpful in chronic recurrent urticaria, whether the psychological disturbance is a primary aggravating factor or secondary to the condition.

13

ERYTHEMA MULTIFORME

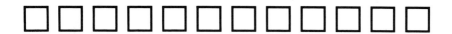

INTRODUCTION

Erythema multiforme is probably an immunological disorder, the end-result being a vasculitis in the skin and mucous membranes. Fifty per cent of cases arise spontaneously, the remainder following a variety of precipitating factors, including drugs, infections – particularly herpes simplex and mycoplasma – and pregnancy. As the name implies, the morphology of the eruption is extremely variable. The condition may occur at any age but is commoner in children and young adults.

CLINICAL FEATURES

Classically the initial lesion is an erythematous macule which becomes papular or blistering (Figure 24) and then extends peripherally with central clearing; as the border extends, new lesions appear at the centre, setting up a series of rings – so forming the 'iris' or target lesion. The secondary central lesions are occasionally purpuric. Often, however, the rash is not classical but greatly varied – with macules, papules, urticaria, purpura and blistering lesions occurring either singly or in combination.

The rash is symmetrical and commonly on backs and fronts of hands. Occasionally the lesions are widespread, extending to trunk and limbs and becoming confluent. In the severe form of the disorder known as the Stevens–Johnson syndrome there is involvement of the mouth, eyes and genitalia. Upper respiratory lesions may lead to difficulties with ventilation and swallowing, and eye lesions may progress to iritis, uveitis or even panophthalmitis.

PROBLEMS AND MANAGEMENT

Diagnosis may be difficult, owing to polymorphism of the eruption. Bullous erythema multiforme can be especially difficult to distinguish from pemphigoid, and biopsy with immunofluorescent study may be required.

Besides the problems of diagnosis it is important to realize that the severity of the condition may vary enormously. Mild cases are often asymptomatic, clear in 2–3 weeks, and require no treatment. Moderate cases may be associated with constitutional disturbance such as fever, headache, and arthralgia, the patient requiring bed-rest and, if the rash is irritating, oral antihistamines. Severe cases such as the potentially fatal Stevens–Johnson syndrome often require intensive care and systemic steroids.

Another point to bear in mind when assessing the condition is that some patients go on to develop recurrent episodes of erythema multiforme, the intervals between attacks varying from a few weeks to a few years.

Efforts must be made to identify possible precipitating causes. Drugs, especially sulphonamides and barbiturates, may be responsible, and if so, should be stopped and never taken again. Viral infections, particularly herpes simplex, may trigger off the condition, as may mycoplasma, streptococcal and meningococcal infections. Radiotherapy in the treatment of malignancy has also been implicated as precipitating some cases of erythema multiforme.

14

BENIGN NEOPLASMS

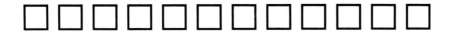

These may be classified as follows:

(1)   Pigmented naevi

(2)   Juvenile melanoma

(3)   Seborrhoeic warts

(4)   Skin tags

(5)   Milia (keratin cysts)

(6)   Keratoacanthoma

(7)   Histiocytomata

(8)   Keloids

(9)   Congenital haemangiomata

(10)   Acquired haemangiomata

(11)   Hereditary telangiectasia

(12)   Lymphangiomata

(13)   Other lesions derived from skin appendages

PIGMENTED NAEVI

Introduction

Naevus is the Latin word for 'mole' and literally means 'blemish' or 'lump' on the skin, and therefore may be used to describe any lump or bump on the skin. 'Pigmented' naevi are considered a separate group as they are all derived from melanocytes.

Pigmented naevi can be typed by either histological or clinical description. Histologically the melanocytes undergo a variable degree of change and may migrate. If they remain in the base of the epidermis they form the 'junctional' nacvus; if the cells migrate both into epidermis and dermis they form the 'compound' naevus, and if they migrate entirely into the dermis they form the 'intradermal' naevus. Only the cells in the epidermis have a potential for malignant change. Intradermal naevi may stop producing melanin, causing a non-pigmented lesion.

Pigmented naevi are present in 95% of white people and should not be considered an abnormality, but rather as a variation of normal cutaneous reaction. The main aetiological factors implicated are heredity, hormones and sunlight. Pigmented naevi are not all present at birth and may appear in infancy and childhood. They seem to be hormone-dependent, as they may arise for the first time at puberty, during pregnancy or in women taking the contraceptive pill.

Clinical features

Pigmented naevi may be (1) flat, (2) slightly raised, (3) sessile and dome-shaped, or (4) 'epidermal' or 'warty'. The flat type and 'junctional' may be extensive, and are commonest on palms and soles. The slightly raised type are often hairy, and histologically 'compound'. The sessile or dome-shaped type are also often hairy and may be very numerous; histologically they are predominantly intradermal.

Naevi of the epidermal type are not true pigmented naevi as they do not arise from melanocytes, although they are associated with increased melanocytic activity; in fact they arise from keratino-cytes; clinically, the lesions are raised, warty (rough surface with clefts), often linear and occasionally extensive.

Other clinically distinct types of pigmented naevi which are variants within the above groups are Becker's hairy epidermal naevus, the halo naevus and the blue naevus.

Problems

Pigmented naevi are very common and malignant change is very rare. However, malignancy should be suspected if there are any of the following features:

(1)   sudden enlargement,

(2)   development of satellite pigmented lesions,

(3)   alteration in pigmentation of the lesion or surrounding skin, either increase or decrease,

(4)   bleeding or ulceration of the lesion,

(5)   the very rare congenital pigmented naevus which is often large, raised and irregular, possesses an intrinsic risk for malignant change and also may be associated with other severe developmental abnormalities, such as spina bifida.

Management

As described above, any suspicion of malignancy necessitates removal of the lesion. Otherwise excision is for cosmetic reasons, or because the lesion is prominent and subject to trauma.

JUVENILE MELANOMA

This implies a naevus which appears in childhood and grows rapidly, but it is always benign. Pigmented naevi generally do not undergo malignant change prior to puberty.

SEBORRHOEIC WARTS

These lesions are not 'viral' warts, but look 'warty'. They are common in the middle-aged and elderly, usually occurring on the face or trunk. The lesions are round, slightly raised, and pigmented (Figure 25), and have a cleft surface and greasy appearance. Initially they may grow rapidly, but they do not become malignant. They can be removed for cosmetic reasons by curettage and cautery.

SKIN TAGS

These are common in the middle-aged, mostly occurring around the neck and in the axillae. They are fibro-epithelial polyps and can be easily removed by snipping the base with scissors and then cauterizing.

MILIA (KERATIN CYSTS)

These are small (1–2mm) whitish yellow papules that usually occur on the face, around the eyes, but may also arise in areas of previously damaged skin, usually following blisters. The lesions are common, mostly in females, and are seen at any age; they are thought to originate from maldeveloped sweat or sebaceous glands. The lesions may be confused with xanthelasma around the eyes, but these usually enlarge to form plaques. Milia do not resolve spontaneously and can be treated for cosmetic reasons with the point of a scalpel blade by breaking the epidermis, and piercing and extruding the cyst.

KERATOACANTHOMA

This is a papule that grows rapidly over a period of 3 months, developing a rolled edge and central crater filled with a keratin plug. The condition remains static for 3 months and then involutes over the next 3 months. Because of its rapid growth and ulcerated appearance a biopsy is often required to exclude malignancy, but once the diagnosis is established the lesion can be left. If treatment is required for cosmetic reasons, curettage and cautery provide the simplest approach.

HISTIOCYTOMATA

These are fairly common benign dermal lesions usually occurring on the lower legs, perhaps following trauma. They are more common in women. Lesions are firm, nodular (0.5–2 cm diameter), and smooth due to overlying epidermis being unaffected. The only treatment is surgical excision, if patients want them removed, but they can be left and there is no tendency to malignant change.

KELOIDS

These lesions result from an abnormal response of dermal connective tissue to trauma, although in Asians and Negroes keloids can occur spontaneously, usually on the trunk. The most effective treatment is intralesional steroid injection as early as possible. Other treatments include radiotherapy after surgical excision, and cryotherapy.

CONGENITAL HAEMANGIOMATA (STRAWBERRY AND PORTWINE)

The two well-known types are the 'strawberry naevus', which is rarely present at birth and usually appears in the first week of life, and the 'portwine stain' which is present to full extent ('mature') at birth. The strawberry naevus may continue growing for up to 18 months; after 3 years the naevus usually shrinks and becomes paler and should disappear by the age of 5 or 6 years, though occasionally there is some residual puckering or scarring. The portwine stain may be extensive and a severe cosmetic problem. Masking creams are the only real help, although some centres are now researching the use of laser therapy. So far the best results are obtained in adults as opposed to children.

ACQUIRED HAEMANGIOMATA

The pyogenic granuloma is a common acquired haemangioma and a misnomer because the lesion was originally thought to be due to a staphylococcal infection. The 'granuloma' usually presents as a solitary, raised, red, variably sized papule (Figure 26) which bleeds on the slightest contact. The most effective treatment is curettage and cautery under local anaesthetic.

Campbell de Morgan spots and spider naevi are other common acquired haemangiomata. The latter are occasionally multiple and associated with pregnancy or liver disease; treatment, if required, is usually by cautery to the central red papule.

HEREDITARY TELANGIECTASIA

This is a rare disease seen as small haemangiomata on face, lips and tongue, the importance of recognizing the condition being due to the fact that the lesions also occur throughout the gastrointestinal tract and may give rise to severe haemorrhage.

LYMPHANGIOMATA

These are rare lesions presenting as grouped deep blisters from which fluid can easily be expressed. If surgically excised they tend to recur. The best cosmetic results are obtained by light cautery.

OTHER LESIONS DERIVED FROM SKIN APPENDAGES

These include tumours of hair follicle and sweat gland origin, the latter being called a syringoma; also the dermal cylindroma, leiomyoma, sebaceous naevus, glomus tumour, and the mast cell tumours of urticaria pigmentosa. All these conditions are rare.

15

SKIN MALIGNANCY

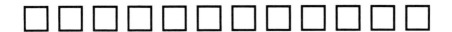

Skin malignancies may be classified as follows:

(1) Basal cell epithelioma
(2) Squamous cell epithelioma
(3) Malignant melanoma
(4) Intraepidermal epithelioma
(5) Senile or actinic keratosis
(6) Skin reticulosis
(7) Secondary carcinoma

BASAL CELL EPITHELIOMA

Introduction

This is the commonest malignant tumour of the skin and is also known as basal cell carcinoma or 'rodent ulcer'. It usually occurs on the face, commonly below eyes or beside the nose. The lesion appears to be induced by ultraviolet light, especially in fair-skinned people and although mostly seen in the middle-aged and elderly, it may occur in younger people – who are then usually of European descent and have had much exposure to strong sunlight in places like South Africa and Australia.

Clinical features

Commonly the lesion begins as a small papule which then spreads outwards leaving a central ulcer (Figure 27). Characteristic telangiectasia may be seen in the raised and pearl-coloured edges. The lesion may ulcerate and bleed, and form a persistent scab, and if left untreated gradually enlarge in annular fashion. Occasionally, there is no ulceration, leaving the cystic or nodular (Figure 28) type which has an irregular surface with telangiectasia. Other less common types are the fibrotic morphoeic form, pigmented types, and superficial types, seen on the trunk.

Management

Biopsy, or excision biopsy if feasible, should be ideally carried out in all cases, and treatment must be carried out by a specialist if possible. The basal cell epithelioma is slow growing and does not metastasize, so the prognosis, if treatment is early, is good. For lesions less than 1 cm in diameter, curettage and cautery provide a 90% cure rate; although the recurrence rate is higher than with surgery or radiotherapy, the cosmetic result is usually better. Radiotherapy, which tends to be reserved for the elderly patient, will probably cause scarring and telangiectasia at the site of the treated lesion 5–10 years later. Excision is often the treatment of choice in the younger patient with lesions greater than 1 cm in diameter. The superficial spreading lesions which occur on the trunk may be treated with curettage and cautery even if extensive. The lesions do not tend to invade deeply.

SQUAMOUS CELL EPITHELIOMA

The skin tumour also occurs in exposed areas but most commonly on backs of hands, pinnae, and lips (Figure 29), and it may also develop on the tongue. In addition to sunlight, chronic trauma and chronic inflammation are considered to be aetiological factors, and the tumour may arise at the site of some chronic skin disorders such as discoid lupus erythematosus.

The epithelioma begins as a small nodule which may ulcerate with rolled edges, or form a scabbed nodule; on the lip the lesion may present as a persistent fissure or ulcer. Early diagnosis, with biopsy confirmation, and early treatment by surgery and/or radiotherapy are essential in order to avoid metastases.

MALIGNANT MELANOMA

This is a relatively rare skin tumour that may occur anywhere on the body. It is not known how many lesions arise *de novo* and how many develop in pre-existing pigmented naevi (see Problems section under Pigmented Naevi, p. 93, for suspicious changes occurring in moles). The incidence of malignant melanoma has increased fourfold over the past two decades, probably due to increased exposure to ultraviolet rays.

The tumour is rare before puberty and develops at any time in adult life. The lesion is irregular, variably pigmented, and *grows rapidly* and irregularly; it may be nodular, ulcerated, scabbed or plaque-like (Figure 30).

Treatment of malignant melanoma is usually by surgery with wide excision and skin graft. If the lesion is large and diagnosis in doubt, initial biopsy is justified. Radiotherapy is sometimes used for primary lesions if they are very large and the patient elderly. Excision of regional lymph nodes is only carried out if there is clinical involvement. Immunotherapy and chemotherapy have been used for both primary and widespread disease. The rate of spread and development of secondary deposits is unpredictable and makes prognosis difficult, although nodular lesions have a poorer prognosis than plaque ones.

INTRAEPIDERMAL EPITHELIOMATA

This implies 'carcinoma *in situ*', the well-known lesions being Bowen's disease, Paget's disease of the breast and erythroplasia of Queyrat of the penis. Bowen's disease presents as a persistent, slow growing, erythematous scaly plaque (Figure 31) that may remain non-invasive and confined to the epidermis for years before changing to a squamous cell epithelioma. Diagnosis should be confirmed by biopsy and treatments possible are curettage and cautery (for the smaller lesion), excision and graft, radiotherapy, and topical 5-fluorouracil. Paget's disease of the breast, although an intraepidermal carcinoma, is usually part of an intraductal carcinoma and will probably necessitate mastectomy.

SENILE OR ACTINIC KERATOSES

These lesions occur on exposed parts and are not initially malignant but are thought to have the potential to develop into squamous cell epitheliomata at a later date. They are commoner in fair-skinned people living in sunny climates. The lesions are greyish-brown discrete patches with slightly raised crumbling surfaces (Figure 32); the surface may be traumatized, leaving an ulcer. The lesions are usually numerous and best treated by topical 5-fluorouracil, but cryotherapy or cautery may also be used.

SKIN RETICULOSIS

Sarcomata, leukaemia and Hodgkin's disease may manifest as infiltrated papules or plaques in the skin. Mycosis fungoides is a distinct reticulosis that originates in the skin but which eventually may be associated with internal reticulosis. The condition commences at any time from early adult life and presents as persistent erythematous scaly patches that may be mistaken for eczema or psoriasis; these lesions may persist for years before becoming infiltrated nodules which may ulcerate. PUVA therapy is used to clear early lesions, and application of powerful topical steroids suppresses irritation and inflammation. Radiotherapy is required for infiltrated plaques and nodules.

Kaposi's sarcoma is probably a reticulosis, and is of current concern as it can be a feature of AIDS (acquired immune deficiency syndrome). The typical lesions are dark blue, occurring on the foot and around the ankle, initially as macules becoming papular, nodular or plaque-like, and occasionally ulcerating. Lesions may begin on the hands, ears or nose, and foot lesions tend to spread up the leg. Surgery, radiotherapy and cytotoxic drugs have been used but none are curative, and in the elderly (when the disease is not associated with AIDS) the course of the disease tends to be very slow and patients may die of other disorders.

SECONDARY CARCINOMATA

The most common primary cancers to metastasize to skin are breast, kidney and lung. The lesions present as firm nodules and are usually a late manifestation of the disease and a poor prognostic sign, although a hypernephroma may present with a solitary skin deposit and in this case treatment of the primary has a better prognosis. Occasionally, intra-abdominal carcinomata may produce deposits in the umbilicus.

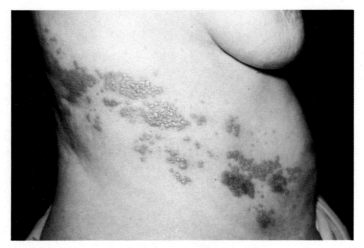

1. Herpes zoster. Blisters confined to area supplied by one sensory nerve.

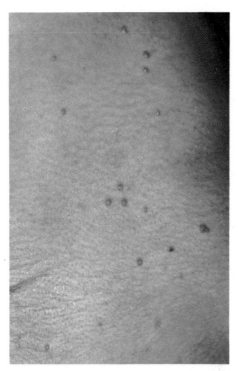

2. Molluscum contagiosum. Pearl coloured papules.

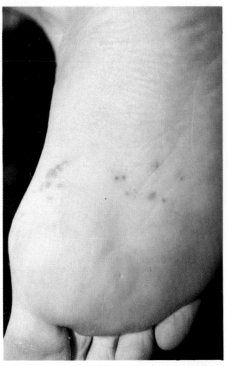

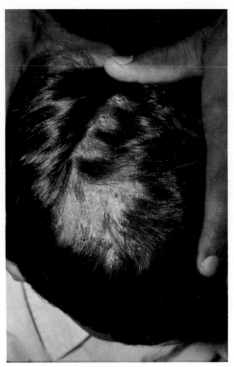

3. Fungal infection of foot, presenting as blisters.

4. Fungal infection of scalp. Scaling is a characteristic feature.

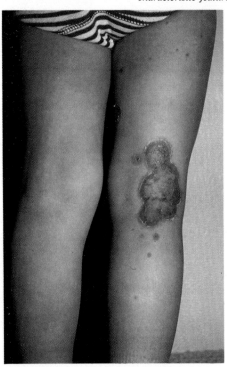

5. Impetigo. Thin roof blisters breaking down to form erosions.

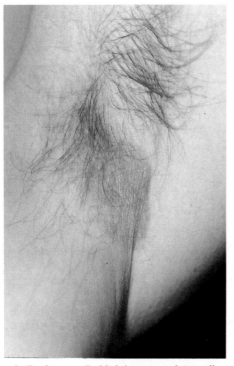

6. Erythrasma. Reddish-brown patch in axilla.

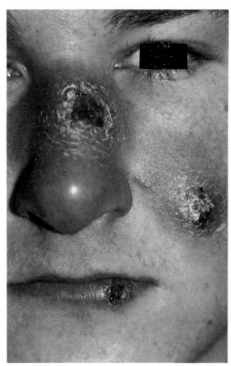

7. Leishmaniasis.

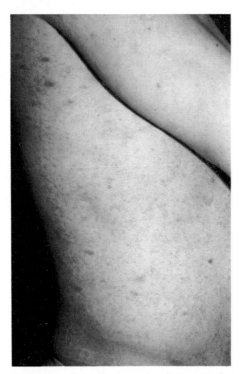

8. Scabies. Generalised eruption. Large papules common on sides of trunk particularly around axillae.

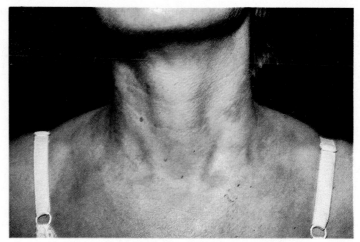

9. Contact eczema on neck from nail varnish.

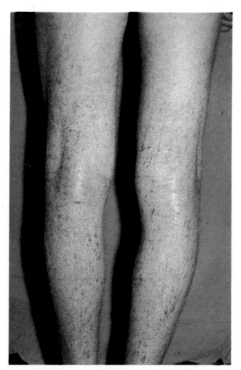

10. Atopic eczema. Excoriated lichenified skin.

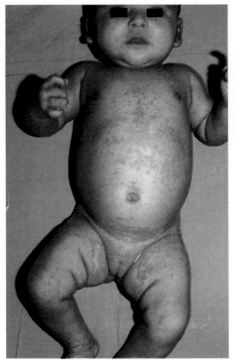

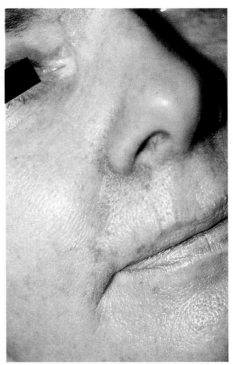

11. Seborrhoeic eczema of infancy, widespread involvement.

12. Seborrhoeic eczema in the naso-labial fold.

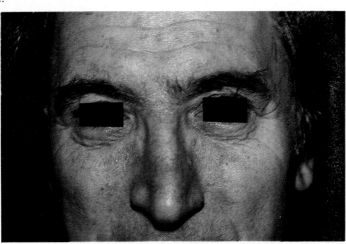

13. Seborrhoeic eczema of forehead and cheeks.

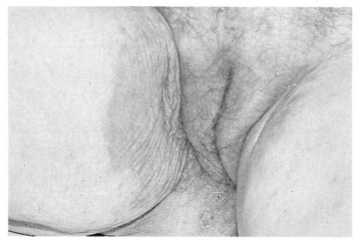

14. Intertrigo, a form of seborrhoeic eczema.

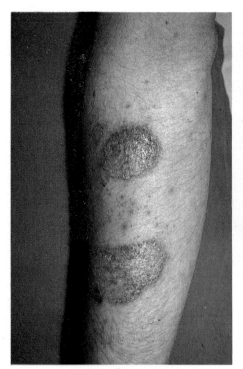

15. Discoid eczema.

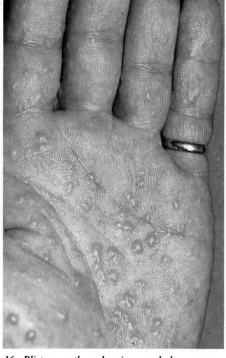

16. Blisters on the palms in pompholyx eczema.

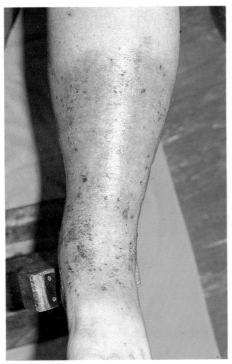

17. *Hypostatic eczema.*

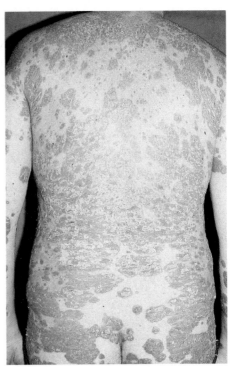

18. *Widespread psoriasis.*

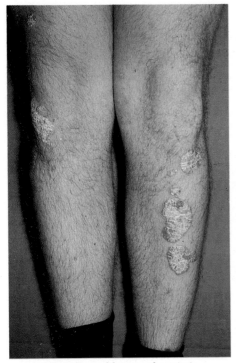

19. *Typical lesions of psoriasis.*

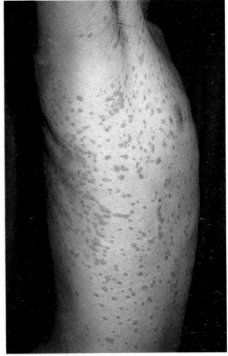

20. *Guttate psoriasis.*

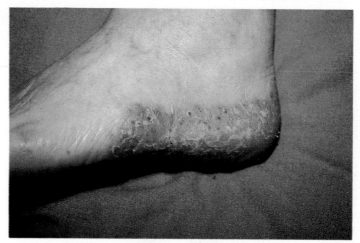

21. Pustular psoriasis.

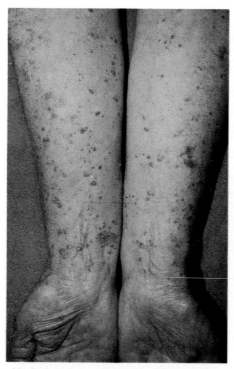

22. Lichen planus. The commonest site is the flexor aspect of the forearms.

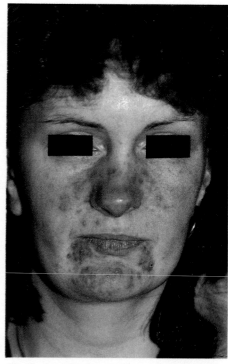

23. Rosacea. Erythema with papules and pustules.

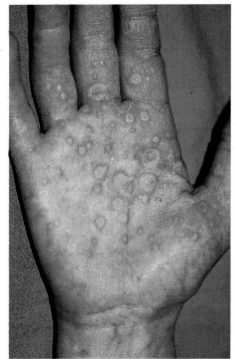

24. Erythema multiforme. The hands are a common site.

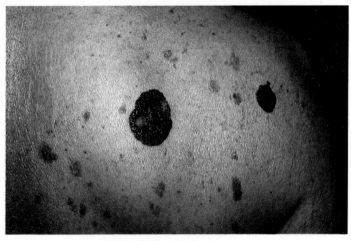

25. Multiple seborrhoeic warts.

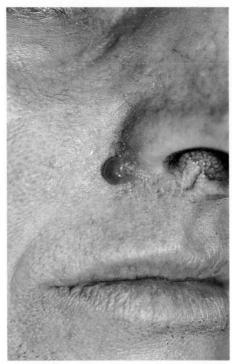

26. Pyogenic granuloma (acquired haemangioma)

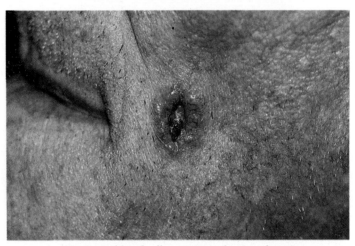

27. Typical basal cell carcinoma, showing ulceration.

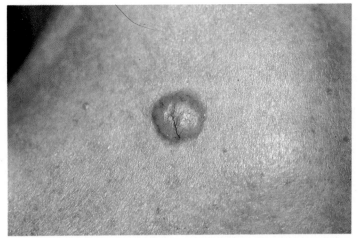

28. Nodular or cystic basal carcinoma. Telangiectasia are frequently present.

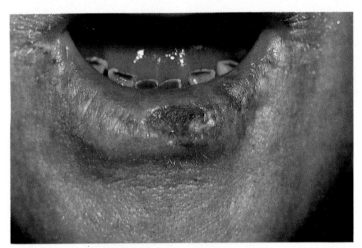

29. Squamous cell carcinoma on the lip.

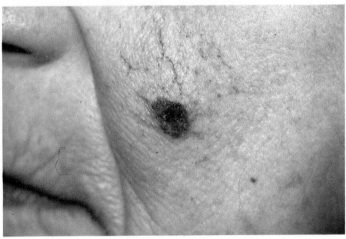

30. Malignant melanoma. Pigmented plaque with irregular surface.

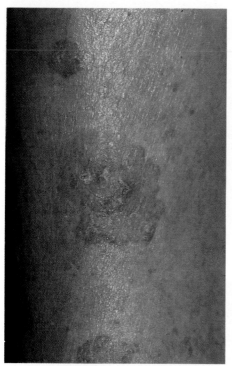

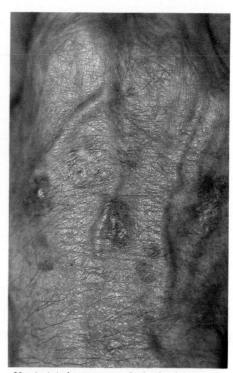

31. *Bowen's disease or intra-epidermal carcinoma.*

32. *Actinic keratoses on the back of the hands.*

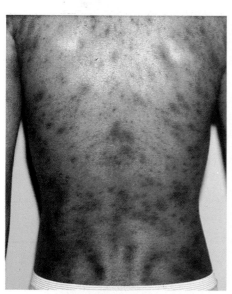

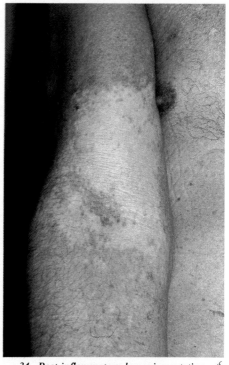

33. *Post-inflammatory hyperpigmentation following a drug rash.*

34. *Post-inflammatory hypopigmentation following eczema.*

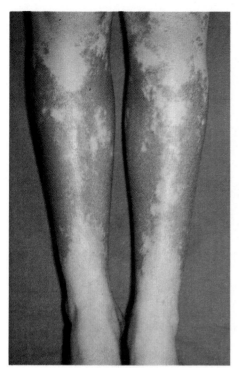

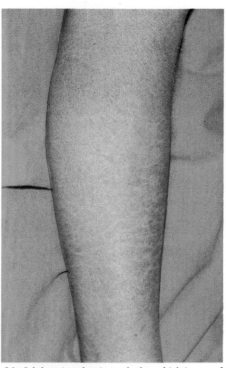

35. *Vitiligo.*

36. *Ichthyosis vulgaris on the leg which is one of the commonest sites.*

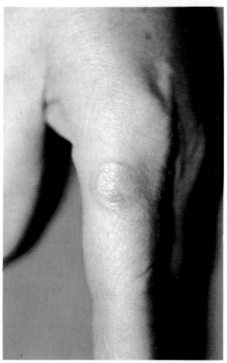

37. *Granuloma annulare.*

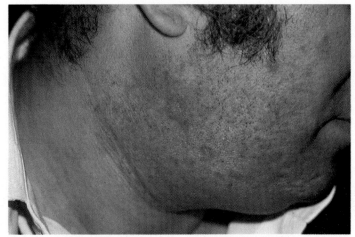

38. Discoid lupus erythematosus showing scarring.

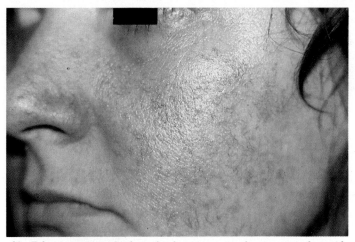

39. Telangiectasia on the face after long term use of potent topical steroids.

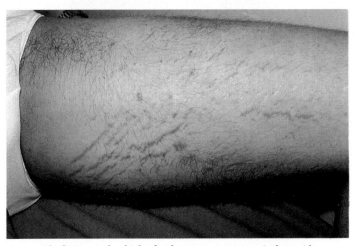

40. Striae on the thigh after long-term potent topical steroids.

16

DISORDERS OF PIGMENTATION

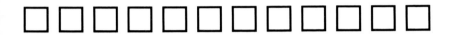

POSTINFLAMMATORY ALTERATION IN PIGMENTATION

Introduction

Inflammatory changes in the skin are a common feature of many skin disorders; similar changes also occur after trauma to the skin particularly after burns. In some instances there is increased pigmentation (Figure 33), whilst in others there is decreased pigmentation (Figure 34). Increased pigmentation may be due to stimulation of melanocytes and/or retention of melanin granules in the upper dermis in macrophages after there has been destruction of the basal layer of the epidermis. Hypopigmentation may be due to inhibition of melanocyte function, loss of melanocytes due to rapid turnover of the epidermis as in psoriasis, or alteration of the keratinocytes in which they are unable to take up melanin granules.

Clinical features

Postinflammatory changes in pigmentation are more likely to occur, and are more apparent, in dark-skinned people, i.e. Asians and Negroes. Hyperpigmentation is most commonly seen in association with eczema, lichen planus, acne and burns. Hypopigmentation is usually found in psoriasis, some forms of eczema, particularly pityriasis alba, discoid lupus erythematosus and syphilis. It can be seen from the above however, that in the same instances a skin disorder will lead to increased pigmentation, whilst in others the same disease may lead to decreased pigmentation in the affected areas.

The alteration in pigmentation tends to localize to the exact sites of the skin disease and may only become apparent once the original skin disorder clears, e.g. as in psoriasis. Occasionally the primary skin disorder may be so mild it goes unnoticed, and the patient presents to the doctor with altered patchy pigmentation; this is particularly common with mild eczema.

The prognosis of postinflammatory altered pigmentation tends to be good and the colour of the skin usually returns to normal once the primary disorder has cleared. However, postinflammatory pigmentation may persist for many months, particularly in Negroes, before fading.

Problems

Postinflammatory hypopigmentation has to be distinguished from pityriasis versicolor particularly when there is involvement of the upper arms, shoulders and upper trunk, and mycological studies may be necessary to distinguish between the two conditions. Vitiligo in its early stages may be similar to postinflammatory hypopigmentation. Eventually vitiligo tends to lead to total loss of pigmentation rather than a partial loss, which tends to occur in postinflammatory changes. Distinction between the two conditions is difficult if there is no preceding history of a previous eruption.

Postinflammatory hyperpigmentation has to be distinguished from melasma (which only occurs on the face, *see below)*, increased pigmentation due to topically applied photosensitizers, e.g. certain perfumes, and systemic drugs which may cause photosensitization, e.g. nalidixic acid, chlorpromazine and tetracyclines. Occasionally patchy pigmentation due to Addison disease may have to be considered in the differential diagnosis.

Assessment and investigation

Usually the diagnosis can be made on the history and the distribution of the eruption. Mycological studies may be necessary in hypopigmented areas on the trunk, and endocrine studies necessary to exclude hypoadrenalism when there are hyperpigmented areas, particularly on the face.

Management

Fortunately the normal colour returns in the majority of patients once the primary disorder has resolved. Hyperpigmentation tends to clear more slowly and occasionally lasts for months. No treatment is usually necessary once the natural history has been explained to the patient.

Referral to specialist

This is only necessary to establish the diagnosis, if in doubt, or to treat the underlying condition, if it is persisting.

VITILIGO

Introduction

Vitiligo is areas of depigmentation due to loss of melanocytes in the affected area. Patients with vitiligo have an increased incidence of organ-specific autoimmune disorders, and increased incidence of autoantibodies even without these disorders. Thus vitiligo is considered to have an autoimmune basis, although as yet, no antibody to melanocytes has been identified.

Clinical features

Vitiligo may present in childhood or adult life; the sexes are equally affected. The lesions are depigmented areas with oval or irregular outline and they tend to extend peripherally. The lesions are usually symmetrical (Figure 35). The common sites of initial involvement are the face, around the eyes and mouth, the axillae and groins, the back of the hands, and extensor surfaces of knees and elbows. However, any area may be involved.

Vitiligo may extend to involve large areas of the skin, either by extension of existing lesions or new lesions developing. Very rarely the whole of the skin may be affected. Alternatively, once the initial lesions have appeared there may be no further involvement of the skin. Vitiligo usually persists but on rare occasions spontaneous remission does occur.

In some instances the hair in the affected areas may become white, but this is not a common feature, and in the majority of patients the melanocytes in the hair follicle remain functional.

Apart from the cosmetic effect of vitiligo the disease is symptomless, unless patients expose the affected areas to sunlight. As the affected areas have no functioning melanocytes or melanin these areas will become red and easily become sunburnt.

Problems

These include the embarrassing appearance of the skin, particularly in Asians and Negroes, and the fact that patients will have to keep the affected areas out of the sun. The other causes of lack of pigmentation that have to be considered are pityriasis versicolor and postinflammatory hypopigmentation. Mycology should distinguish pityriasis versicolor, if there is any doubt, and in postinflammatory hypopigmentation there may well be a history of previous eruption or some change in texture such as scaling may be present.

Assessment and investigation

If the diagnosis is made with certainty, no investigations are necessary. If there is doubt, particularly when there is involvement of the upper trunk, scrapings should be taken for mycology. Although there is an increased incidence of autoimmune disorders in vitiligo, the incidence is still very low (less than 1%) and unless there is clinical evidence of any organ-specific disease, screening tests are not necessary.

Management

The two measures which may reverse the condition are topical steroids and psoralens combined with ultraviolet light (PUVA). Topical steroids are successful in no more than 20% of patients and have to be used for many months, thus there are risks from side-effects, and in vitiligo weak topical steroids are not effective. Psoralens combined with ultraviolet are often successful in over half the patients. A poor prognostic sign is extensive disease. There is some evidence that the darker the normal skin, the better the response to treatment.

If vitiligo affects the face and hands and is causing embarrassment, suitable cosmetic camouflage can hide the lesions. If patients cannot camouflage the lesions themselves they should be referred for expert camouflage advice.

When patients go to a sunny climate they should keep the affected areas covered as much as is practical and use sunscreens to protect the affected areas.

Occasionally if the disease is very extensive and there are only a few normal areas remaining, it is justifiable to depigment these areas, so that the patients have a uniform colour.

Referral to specialist

This is necessary if patients wish for treatment or there is doubt about the diagnosis.

MELASMA (CHLOASMA)

Introduction

This is a common disorder of facial hyperpigmentation, mainly seen in women, particularly in those from the Middle East.

Clinical features

The common areas to be affected are the upper cheeks, upper lip, nose and centre of the forehead. Melasma usually first appears in young adults and middle age. The lesions are pale or dark brown with an irregular border.

In whites, melasma is most often seen during pregnancy and occasionally after taking an oral contraceptive. Although similar events may cause melasma in Asians, it also frequently occurs spontaneously.

Melasma in white people fades after pregnancy or stopping the contraceptive pill, but when it is spontaneous the condition is often persistent. Melasma tends to fade in the winter and darken in the summer. Female hormones appear to be an important aetiological factor even in spontaneous melasma. The condition is rare in postmenopausal women.

Problems

Melasma has to be distinguished from postinflammatory hyper-pigmentation and increased pigmentation from topical photosen-sitizers, particularly those found in cosmetics. Some systemic drugs may also act as photosensitizers and may result in increased pig-mentation. In hypoadrenalism, pigmentation is usually found at other sites, particularly the oral cavity, although it must be remem-bered that in Asians pigmentation in the oral cavity occurs in 40% of individuals.

Investigations

None are usually necessary, but if there is any doubt about hypo-adrenalism then tests for adrenal function must be carried out.

Management

If patients are taking an oral contraceptive, a change to a different form of contraception should be advised. Sunscreens should be used during the summer months to stop the lesions becoming darker and more obvious. A suitable camouflage cosmetic should be advised if patients are embarrassed by their appearance. Topical hydroquinone preparations may lighten the areas but should be used with caution and only for short periods at a time. These preparations should only be used under medical supervision.

LENTIGINES

A lentigo is a small persistent permanent hyperpigmented macule. The commonest cause for a lentigo is ultraviolet light, and they are predominantly seen in white people particularly those who have lived in tropical or semitropical climates. In whites who live in sunny climates they usually appear during the third and fourth decades and then increase in number and size. In persons living in Britain, they are seen in those who pursue outdoor activities, and they tend to appear around middle age. They are a common finding in elderly people who have been sunworshippers in their younger days. If treatment is requested, cryotherapy is often successful in removing the lesions.

Non-actinic lentigines usually appear in childhood and would seem to be a development abnormality of the skin with increased activity of the melanocytes in the affected area.

17

BULLOUS DISORDERS

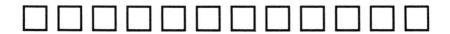

These are a group of disorders in which the predominant skin lesion is a blister.

PEMPHIGUS

Introduction

This is an autoimmune disease characterized by an antibody to the cell membrane of the epidermal cells.

Clinical features

Pemphigus is most commonly seen in the 40–60 age group, although it may occur in both younger and older persons. As the blister in pemphigus is intraepidermal the roof is very thin and thus the blister ruptures easily. The lesions may therefore be flaccid blisters, erosions or crusted areas. The lesions may occur on any part of the body. Initially there may be only a few lesions but, untreated, the disease may be extensive with large weeping areas. Pemphigus also affects the mucous membranes and presents as painful erosions particularly in the mouth. The eyes, nasal mucosa and genitalia may also be involved. Pemphigus may in fact begin in the mouth and stay localized to the oral cavity for months or even years before skin lesions appear.

If untreated, pemphigus is invariably fatal. Before the advent of steroids death usually occurred approximately 2 years after the first lesions appeared.

Problems

Although there are drugs which will now suppress pemphigus there is a high incidence of morbidity and occasionally mortality from these drugs. The mortality from pemphigus and its treatment is still approximately 10%.

The differential diagnosis of pemphigus includes the other bullous disorders, pemphigoid, erythema multiforme, and dermatitis herpetiformis. Erosions are not common in these diseases and the blisters tend to have an urticarial base. Toxic epidermal necrolysis may also present with widespread erosions but the onset is usually sudden. Widespread impetigo may have similar lesions to pemphigus, but usually the onset is more sudden.

The differential diagnosis of the oral lesions includes erosive lichen planus, mucous membrane pemphigoid, Behçet's disease, and persistent aphthous ulcers.

Assessment and investigation

Biopsies of a lesion for routine histology and of perilesional skin for immunofluorescent studies are essential. Routine histology shows an intraepidermal blister and immunofluorescent studies will show deposition of IgG on the surface of the epidermal cells. Blood should also be taken for detection of circulating antibodies against epidermal cell membrane.

Management

Systemic steroids

These form the basis of treatment. The initial dose is 60–120mg per day. The dose is gradually reduced when new lesions stop forming and the old ones begin to heal. However, it is not unusual that patients will have to take a maintenance dose for a considerable length of time (months or even years). The dose will depend on the activity of the disease and there are no objective tests for determining this activity. Eventual remission does occur in pemphigus in a large proportion of patients but this may not be for months or years after the onset. Subsequent recurrence after remission may also occur.

Immunosuppressive drugs

These are used in addition to steroids in an attempt to reduce the amount of steroid required to control the disease. The following have been used: azathioprine, methotrexate, cyclophosphamide, gold and dapsone. There is no agreement as to which one of these drugs is the best.

Plasmapheresis

This has been used when it has been difficult to control the disease with reasonable doses of steroids and immunosuppressive drugs. The results are variable but a number of patients do seem to have benefited.

Complications

The main complication of pemphigus *per se* is secondary infection. However, the main problems currently seen are due to the drugs used to control the disease, and these are principally associated with long-term steroid therapy. Suppression of the bone marrow and increased susceptibility to infections are those more frequently seen due to immunosuppressive drugs.

Referral to specialist

This is essential for diagnosis and management.

Long-term care

This is also usually supervised by the specialist. Patients taking steroids should have their weight, blood pressure and urine checked at regular intervals. A full blood count is necessary at appropriate intervals in patients taking immunosuppressive drugs.

PEMPHIGOID

Introduction

This is an autoimmune disease with the antibody directed against the basement membrane.

Clinical features

Pemphigoid is most commonly seen in the elderly. The typical lesion is a large tense blister on an urticarial base. The eruption is symmetrical and affects the trunk and limbs. The face and scalp are usually spared. The eruption tends to be widespread and presents as large plaques of urticaria. Occasionally prior to the rash patients complain of severe irritation. Pemphigoid tends to be a chronic condition but spontaneous remission does occur in a proportion of patients, although not usually for 2 years. Unlike pemphigus the disease did not usually prove fatal prior to the availability of steroids.

Problems

Because the disorder is frequently widespread and itchy, treatment is necessary, and problems are usually due to the drugs used to suppress the rash.

Assessment and investigation

Patients should be referred for biopsies which will show a sub-epidermal blister and a band of IgG along the line of basement membrane in the perilesional and uninvolved skin.

Management

Systemic steroids are the most effective drugs in suppressing the eruption. The initial dose is usually 60mg daily and should be continued until new lesions no longer appear. The dose is gradually reduced but a maintenance dose is usually necessary; this is judged by the clinical response. In an attempt to lower the amount of steroid required for maintenance purposes, it is usual to give azathioprine in addition to the steroids.

There are few complications of the actual disease apart from secondary infection. Complications, however, are seen due to the prolonged use of systemic steroids and immunosuppression from azathioprine.

Referral to specialist

This is necessary for diagnosis and treatment.

Long-term care

This is needed to regulate the dose of drugs according to the activity of the disease. The weight, blood pressure and urine should be checked at regular intervals. A full blood count is necessary at appropriate intervals if patients are taking azathioprine.

DERMATITIS HERPETIFORMIS

Introduction

The rash in dermatitis herpetiformis is gluten-dependent and there is an associated mild gluten enteropathy.

Clinical features

Dermatitis herpetiformis may present at any age but the commonest age of onset is in late adolescence and early adult life. The characteristic sites to be involved are the extensor surface of the elbows and forearms, buttocks, and extensor surface of the knees. If the disorder is widespread any part of the body may be affected. The typical lesions are small tense blisters situated on an urticarial base. The blisters are often grouped. The eruption in dermatitis herpetiformis is intensely irritating and frequently therefore no blisters are seen but only excoriations at the site of the eruption. Dermatitis herpetiformis is a chronic condition; only 10–20% of patients can expect a spontaneous remission and this is usually after many years.

Problems

Due to the associated enteropathy patients may be suffering from iron or folate deficiency. There is also a relatively high incidence of autoimmune diseases, particularly thyroid disease and pernicious anaemia. Although rare, there is an increased incidence of lymphoma in patients with dermatitis herpetiformis, as occurs in patients with coeliac disease. The other problems encountered are usually related to treatment.

Assessment and investigation

The diagnosis should be confirmed by a biopsy of uninvolved skin which will show deposits of IgA in the dermal papillae. Patients should also have a small intestinal biopsy and a full blood count. It is also advisable to investigate for evidence of iron, folate or B_{12} deficiency. Autoantibody screen should also be carried out and if any autoantibodies are present, this may point to certain disorders in later life.

Management

Drugs

The most effective drug in suppressing the rash is dapsone. The initial dose is 100mg daily and the dose is then altered to find the lowest necessary to control the eruption. The rash will clear within a week or two of starting treatment and recur equally quickly when the dapsone is stopped. If patients are unable to take dapsone then the long-acting sulphonamide, sulphamethoxypyridazine, or sulphapyridine should be used.

Gluten free diet

If strict, this will control the rash and heal the enteropathy. It must be stressed that it takes approximately 6 months before drug requirements are decreased and on average 2 years before patients can manage without drugs. The diet must be considered to be life long.

Complications

The commonest seen are due to dapsone therapy. Dapsone invariably causes haemolysis; if severe this will lead to anaemia. Dapsone may also cause headaches, lethargy and a neuropathy.

Referral to specialist

This is necessary initially for confirmation of the diagnosis and full investigation as detailed above.

Long-term care

As the disease is chronic, long-term care is necessary. If patients take a gluten free diet, once the rash is controlled and the enteropathy healed patients will only need to be seen once or twice a year. A full blood count should be carried out once a year and the urine examined, as there is an increased incidence of autoimmune diabetes. If patients are taking dapsone they probably should be seen twice a year and a blood count performed. Particular attention should be paid to detecting evidence of thyroid disease, pernicious anaemia and possibly lymphoma.

18

HAIR PROBLEMS

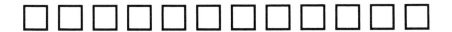

ALOPECIA AREATA

Introduction

This is a very common condition accounting for 2% of new atten-
dances at skin clinics in the UK. The cause of the condition is
unknown but there is some evidence that it has an autoimmune
basis.

Clinical features

Any age may be affected but the condition is rare in the elderly and
in infancy. Alopecia areata usually presents as one or several
circumscribed patches of hair loss. The skin in the affected area is
smooth and non-scaly, and may be slightly erythematous. At the
periphery of the bald area, 'exclamation mark' hairs may be seen.
These are short hairs, usually 5mm in length, which are thicker at
the distal end and taper towards the surface of the scalp. If they are
plucked by forceps they are easily detached from the scalp and the
hair bulb is attached to the end of the hair. Thus the hair and bulb
give the appearance of an exclamation mark. If the disease is
severe, several new patches may appear in a short space of time

and coalesce to form large bald areas. When the scalp above the ears and at the back is involved, this tends to imply a poor prognosis. Occasionally all the hair from the scalp may be lost – so-called alopecia totalis.

Alopecia areata not infrequently begins in the beard area in men, and there may be no involvement of the scalp. Similarly only the eyebrows may be affected. In rare instances all the hair from the body and eyelashes is lost – so-called alopecia universalis. As a general rule, the more extensive the hair loss, the worse the prognosis.

An unusual presentation of alopecia areata is a diffuse hair loss with no bald patches. The name is totally unsuitable for this form of the disorder.

Unless exclamation mark hairs are present it is difficult to distinguish it from other causes of diffuse hair loss. Occasionally the nails are affected in alopecia areata. They tend to be ridged and flaky and occasionally pits are present.

The prognosis of alopecia areata is usually good, and in the majority of patients the hair will regrow spontaneously after a few months. As mentioned above, when the disorder is extensive the prognosis tends to be poor.

Problems

The main problem is the cosmetic disability, and patients may have to wear a wig when the hair loss is extensive. Not surprisingly anxiety and reactive depression may occur.

The differential diagnosis includes fungal infection of the scalp and trichotillomania (pulling or breaking the hair as a habit) in children. Scarring alopecia is easy to distinguish as the skin is not normal.

Assessment and investigation

No tests are necessary if the diagnosis is made on clinical grounds. If there is any scaling of the scalp, fungal infections must be excluded by taking hair and skin for mycological examination.

Management

If only one or two small solitary patches are present, simple re-assurance is all that is necessary. If the patches are large and causing embarrassment, in some patients potent topical steroids do seem to be helpful. Intralesional steroids given with the Dermojet (injecting under pressure) may well speed the regrowth of hair. Other treatments which are currently in vogue and do appear to stimulate regrowth of hair include ultraviolet light, PUVA, topical 1% minoxidil cream, and painting the affected areas with dini-trochlorbenzene. The last treatment should be supervised by a consultant dermatologist. Although systemic steroids are effective it is doubtful whether their use can be justified.

FEMALE CONSTITUTIONAL ALOPECIA

Introduction

Hair loss in women is a common presenting symptom in a skin clinic. The cause for this type of hair loss is not known and thus it is often referred to as constitutional. It has been suggested that this hair loss is androgen dependent, as in men, but there are no other virilizing signs to suggest excess production of androgens. Thus it is assumed that the cause may be an end-organ (in this case the hair root) hypersensitivity disorder to normal levels of androgens. Another theory is that the hair loss may depend on an androgen/oestrogen ratio, and thus after the menopause, when this pattern of hair loss is common, and when oestrogens fall, there may be a relative increase in androgen.

Clinical features

Female constitutional alopecia may occur as early as the third decade, and thereafter may begin at any age. Thinning of the hair is frequent after the menopause, but it is not always severe or obvious in many individuals. Characteristically the top of the scalp is where the thinning occurs and the back and sides of the scalp are often not affected, unless the condition is severe, but these sites are always less affected than the crown. Unlike male pattern alopecia, the condition produces no recession of the fronto-temporal hair line. In addition, unlike male pattern baldness, constitutional hair loss in women does not lead to complete baldness, although in some women the hair may be very thin.

Problems

Although this type of hair loss cannot be considered as a disease, the condition does lead to a great deal of mental anguish. The condition has to be differentiated from telogen effluvium in which the hair loss is reversible. Alopecia due to drugs, thyroid or iron deficiency, and diffuse alopecia areata have also to be considered.

Assessment and investigation

A full history of any recent illnesses, pregnancies and drug intake must be taken. It is probably justifiable to have a full blood count and serum iron and thyroid function estimated to exclude these treatable causes for hair loss. If there are any virilizing features, investigation is necessary to exclude endocrine disorders.

Management

Unfortunately there is no simple safe treatment currently available to reverse female constitutional hair loss. Patients should be reassured that although their hair will remain thin it will not lead to complete baldness. Claims have been made for antiandrogens in premenopausal women and oestrogens in postmenopausal women, but as the condition will revert to its previous state when these drugs are stopped, it is probably inadvisable to prescribe them. It should be left to the discretion of the patient whether she wishes to wear a wig.

Referral to specialist

A second opinion is often asked for in premenopausal women and this seems a reasonable request even if it is only for simple reassurance and exclusion of other causes of hair loss.

TELOGEN EFFLUVIUM

Introduction

Telogen is that part of the hair cycle in which hair stops growing and is shed. It has been estimated that a normal individual may lose fifty hairs per day. In telogen effluvium, however, when a large number of hair follicles enter the resting phase anywhere from 100 to 1000 hairs may be lost daily. The most common cause of telogen effluvium is the postpregnancy state; it is also seen after acute febrile illness, haemorrhage and stopping the contraceptive pill. What actually causes an increased number of hairs to enter the resting phase is unknown but, in view of the above conditions associated with it, there may be hormonal causes.

Clinical features

Usually 2–4 months after the trigger factor the patients begin to notice increase shedding of the hair in a brush, or in the basin after washing. Subsequently, if the condition continues the patient becomes aware of thinning of the hair on the scalp. The hair loss is diffuse and is not confined to any particular part of the scalp. The condition does not lead to complete baldness and is self-limiting although it may persist for up to 1 year. The ultimate prognosis is good, the hair eventually growing to the same quantity as before.

Problems

The condition has to be distinguished from female constitutional alopecia and a diffuse form of alopecia areata.

Assessment and investigation

If the diagnosis can be made with certainty, no investigations are necessary. If there is doubt, iron deficiency and hypothyroidism should be excluded.

Management

There is no treatment which will shorten the duration of hair loss. However, patients should be reassured that the eventual outlook is good and the hair will regrow.

MALE PATTERN ALOPECIA

Introduction

This pattern of hair loss is considered to be normal and not a disease although young male adults frequently seek medical advice for the problem. The cause of this pattern of hair loss is multifactorial, with genetic factors being important.

Clinical features

It is not always appreciated that male pattern hair loss may begin in the late teens. As a general rule, the earlier the hair loss begins, the more severe the condition is likely to be. The first sign is recession of the fronto-temporal hair line. This is followed by gradual thinning of the hair of the posterior vertex. There is considerable variation in the degree of hair loss and the speed with which the hair loss occurs. In the severest form, all the hair is lost apart from the back and sides of the scalp, and this state may be reached even by the early twenties. In other instances the loss may be gradual over many years and the hair becomes thin over the vertex with mild fronto-temporal recession.

Problems

Male pattern alopecia has to be distinguished from telogen effluvium and a diffuse form of alopecia areata. In the latter two conditions the fronto-temporal hair line does not recede.

Management

Patients should be told that there is no effective remedy for male pattern alopecia, and that it should not be considered an abnormality.

Referral to specialist

This is sometimes necessary as the individual wants a second opinion that a treatable disorder is not being missed.

TRICHOTILLOMANIA

Introduction

Trichotillomania is the name given to the condition in which patients present with hair loss due to the hair being broken from self-induced trauma. The hair may be broken by continual rubbing, twisting or pulling of the hair. In some individuals it seems the trauma is inflicted subconsciously and the condition simply appears to be a habit. In others the hair is damaged consciously and in these individuals there may be an underlying psychiatric disorder.

Presentation

The condition is commoner in females, and the commonest age of presentation is in the 5–10 years age group. The patient usually presents with a patch of hair loss. Examination shows hairs to be present in the affected area, but they are broken close to the surface. Careful examination shows the hairs to be of different lengths. The skin appears normal. Occasionally the eyebrows and eyelashes are traumatized in a similar manner and patients present with patchy or total involvement in one or both eyebrows.

Problems

Trichotillomania has to be distinguished from other causes of patchy hair loss. In fungal infections there is scaling of the scalp, and in alopecia areata the hair loss is complete.

Management

If the hair is traumatized as a subconscious habit, attention has to be directed to trying to break the habit. If parents are present they should dissuade the child from the practice. Shaving of the scalp or occlusive bandages to the scalp have been suggested in extreme cases to break the habit. Frequently the children grow out of the practice without any special remedies. If the condition is severe and persistent, however, psychiatric assessment is probably necessary.

Referral to specialist

This is necessary if the diagnosis is in doubt or the condition is severe and shows no signs of spontaneous remission.

HIRSUTISM

Introduction

Hirsutism is the change of soft vellous hair to coarse terminal hair in female subjects. Hirsutism is usually divided into primary and secondary.

In primary hirsuties no underlying endocrine cause is found. The most common cause is racial and the condition is very frequent in persons from the Middle East, Indian subcontinent and Southern Mediterranean countries. So-called idiopathic hirsutism is seen in individuals who have no genetic or underlying endocrine cause. It is thought that in these individuals the fault is one of the end-organ (the hair follicle) in which there is increased sensitivity to normal levels of circulating androgens.

Secondary hirsutism is seen in conditions associated with increased production of androgens, e.g. polycystic ovaries, Cushing disease, congenital adrenal syndrome, arrhenoblastoma and adrenal rest tumour. A number of drugs including anabolic steroids and some progesterones may also cause hirsutism. Hypertrichosis (which is terminal hairs all over the face) may be seen with the hypotensive agents minoxidil and diazoxide.

Presentation

The common sites for hirsutism are the upper lip, chin, lower abdomen from the umbilicus to the pubis, around the nipples, centre of the chest, sacral region, and the arms and legs. Hirsutism often begins around puberty and gradually increases and is fully established by the mid-twenties. There are considerable variations

129

in the degrees of hirsutism, and in some individuals it may simply be an increase of terminal hairs on the limbs, whilst in others it is severe at all the above-mentioned sites.

Assessment and investigations

A detailed menstrual history and full medical examination are necessary. If secondary hirsutism is suspected full endocrinological assessment is necessary. Serum testosterone, sex hormone binding globulin, prolactin and gonadotrophin levels are necessary. Ultrasound examination of the ovaries may also be indicated. These investigations are best supervised by an endocrinologist.

Management

If a secondary cause is found then obviously this should be treated accordingly. However, even if successful this treatment does not always cause regression of the hirsutism once it is established.

In primary hirsutism, and in secondary hirsutism if the hair persists despite treatment of the primary cause, the hair may be removed by waxing or shaving. However, the only permanent method of removal is electrolysis. This is a time-consuming procedure and needs to be carried out by an expert. If the condition is mild, bleaching of the hair may be sufficient for the patient.

Antiandrogen treatment of hirsutism is sometimes indicated if the condition is severe and extensive. The drug used is cyproterone acetate 50–100mg daily during days 5–14 of the menstrual cycle. The drug has to be given with oestrogens, taken during days 5–26 of the cycle. The dose of ethinyl oestradiol is 20–50μg daily. Treatment results in less growth and thinning of the terminal hair in the abnormal sites. However, treatment has to be considered indefinite.

Referral to specialist

This is necessary for full investigation and assessment if the condition is severe and secondary hirsutism is suspected.

19

PHOTOSENSITIVITY

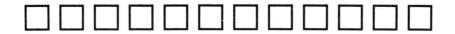

Abnormal reactions to light may either be due to substances applied to the skin (exogenous) or arise from internal (endogenous) causes.

EXOGENOUS PHOTOSENSITIVE ERUPTIONS

Introduction

Exogenous photosensitizers include chemicals found in plants, cosmetics, antibacterial preparations and drugs and from industrial processes.

Presentation

Patients of any age may be affected but because of the substances causing the eruption the condition is more commonly seen in adults. The site of the eruption will depend on where the photosensitizer was applied and whether it was an exposed area. The appearance of the eruption depends on the chemical, as different substances cause different reactions in the skin. Perfumes tend to cause erythema and increased pigmentation on the sides of the neck. This is usually due to a chemical called oil of bergamot which contains psoralens. Chemicals from plants often cause a severe reaction with blisters. If the chemical causing the eruption can be identified and avoided, the prognosis is good. The pigmentation following involvement with oil of bergamot may take months to fade.

Problems

Once it is determined that the eruption is photosensitive, the differential diagnosis is that of the endogenous photosensitive disorders. Occasionally endogenous eczema, particularly atopic, may be made worse by sunlight. Contact eczema which is not photosensitive may give a similar picture, particularly if it is due to substances applied to the face, or if the contact eczema is due to airborne substances.

Assessment and investigation

If the source and identity of the offending substance can be determined on the history, no further action is necessary. If not, then patch tests and photo-patch tests will be necessary. In photo-patch tests the chemicals are applied to the skin and the area irradiated with an artificial light source.

Management

If the disorder is due to an isolated event (e.g. contact from plants in the country) the condition may well settle by itself without treatment. As the reaction in the skin is an inflammatory one, the most appropriate treatment is corticosteroids. If the reaction is very acute, weak topical steroid cream (e.g. 1% hydrocortisone) should be applied four times a day. If blisters are present, normal saline soaks or potassium permanganate soaks 1:8000 (not for the face) should be used for 15 minutes four times daily. Systemic steroids are only indicated if the reaction is very severe or very widespread. The initial dose is prednisone 30mg daily, and this should be reduced as soon as improvement occurs. Patients should be told not to go into the sun until their eruption has settled. Specific advice about avoidance of the offending substance should be given.

Referral to specialist

This is only necessary for identification of the offending substance if not apparent from the history, or if the reaction is very severe and further advice on management is needed.

ENDOGENOUS PHOTOSENSITIVE ERUPTIONS

Photosensitive reactions due to internal causes can be divided into those (1) due to drugs, (2) forming part of a systemic disorder and (3) which are idiopathic, in which there is an abnormal response to light for which there is no known external chemical or internal disease.

DRUG-INDUCED PHOTOSENSITIVITY

Introduction

The drugs which most commonly cause photosensitivity are nalidixic acid, phenothiazines, sulphonamides, tetracyclines and thiazides. However it should be remembered that other drugs may also cause photosensitive reactions.

Clinical features

The eruption occurs on exposed areas of the skin with characteristic sparing of the upper eyelids, under the nose, and neck under the chin. The rash may be erythematous and scaly or in the more severe reactions urticarial and/or bullous. Residual hyperpigmentation may occur particularly with phenothiazines.

An unusual photosensitive reaction seen with tetracyclines is photo-onycholysis, in which the distal half of the nails separates from the nail bed. This may be associated with pain in the fingertips.

The prognosis of photosensitive drug eruptions is good, if the drug is identified and can be stopped. Residual hyperpigmentation may take time to fade.

Problems

It is important to stop the drug that is suspected of causing the photosensitivity. It should also be remembered that each drug in a similar group, e.g. phenothiazines and thiazides, may cause the same reaction, and so if possible a completely different group of drugs should be used.

The differential diagnosis includes photosensitive reactions from topically applied substances and the group of idiopathic photosensitive disorders. Porphyria and lupus erythematosus must also be considered; it should be remembered that both these disorders may be precipitated by drugs. In the case of lupus erythematosus, those responsible are usually hydralazine, penicillin and procainamide, and in porphyria (i.e. that associated with photosensitivity) they are oestrogens, barbiturates, griseofulvin and sulphonamides.

Assessment and investigation

If the diagnosis can be made with certainty no investigations are necessary; if not, tests may have to be carried out to exclude systemic lupus erythematosus and porphyria.

136

Management

If possible the drug should be identified and stopped. If there is any doubt when patients are receiving many different drugs, those most likely to be the cause should be stopped. If a particular drug is thought necessary for long-term use, a substitute should be found. It is important to remember that drugs with similar chemical structure may also be likely to cause the same reaction in an individual. Obviously patients should be kept out of sunlight as much as possible until the rash clears. If there are severe inflammatory changes in the skin, moderate-strength topical steroid creams may be helpful.

Referral to specialist

If the drug causing the photosensitivity can be identified and stopped no referral is necessary.

PHOTOSENSITIVITY DUE TO SYSTEMIC DISORDERS

Systemic lupus erythematosus

This is discussed in Chapter 27.

Porphyria

Introduction

The porphyrias are a group of metabolic disorders in which, due to enzyme abnormalities, there is overproduction of porphyrins. Porphyria is usually inherited but may be acquired in liver damage, the most common cause of which is alcohol. The names given to the porphyrias associated with photosensitivity are partly due to where the excess porphyrin production occurs and partly due to the clinical features (Table 19.1).

Table 19.1   Porphyrias associated with photosensitivity

Name	Inherited or acquired	Onset	Type of lesion	Specimen where porphyria elevation occurs		
				Blood	Urine	Faeces
Congenital erythropoietic	Inherited	Infancy	Blisters and erythema	↑	↑	↑
Erythrohepatic protoporphyria	Inherited	Infancy	Erythema and oedema	↑	–	↑
Porphyria variegate	Inherited	Adolescence	Erosions, blisters crusts and scars	–	↑	↑
Prophyria cutanea tarda	Inherited or acquired	Middle & old age	Blisters and scars	–	↑	±↑

Clinical features

Congenital erythropoietic porphyria is very rare. The photosensitivity occurs on the exposed areas soon after birth and is associated with blisters which may lead to scarring. The eyes are photosensitive and this may lead to blindness. In addition there is a haemolytic anaemia. The porphyrins are also deposited in the teeth and bones, which leads to increased fragility. The urine is pink. The prognosis in congenital erythropoietic porphyria is poor and premature death often occurs from the haemolytic anaemia.

Erythrohepatic protoporphyria, although rare is much commoner than congenital erythropoietic porphyria. Erythrohepatic protoporphyria presents in early childhood with erythema and burning in the exposed areas; oedema and urticaria may also occur. Small linear scars form in the exposed skin. Gallstones due to excess biliary excretion of porphyrins may occur. Erythrohepatic protoporphyria persists throughout life.

Porphyria variegate is most commonly seen in the Afrikaaners of South Africa. The condition presents in adolescence or early adult life, with blisters, crust and erosions in light-exposed areas. Scarring occurs. The skin is fragile and there is often associated hirsutism and premature ageing of the skin. Porphyria variegate is associated with systemic disorders which include abdominal pain and neurological and psychiatric disorders. The disease is aggravated by oestrogens, barbiturates, griseofulvin and sulphonamides. The disorder is persistent and death may result from neurological or psychiatric disease.

Porphyria cutanea tarda presents in middle and old age and is commoner in men. In the light-exposed area, there is blistering, scarring and pigmentation. If alcohol can be avoided the prognosis is good; if alcohol intake cannot be stopped the condition may lead to hepatic failure.

Problems

Apart from porphyria cutanea tarda, which may be helped by

abstinence from alcohol, the conditions are persistent and life long. The differential diagnoses are those of other photosensitive conditions.

Assessment and investigation

Porphyrin estimations in the blood, urine and faeces are necessary. Due to the different enzyme abnormalities in the different porphyrias, the porphyrins will be increased in different specimens (Table 19.1). The serum iron is often raised in porphyria cutanea tarda.

Management

Avoidance of sunlight, as much as possible, is the most effective step. Sunscreens (see p.146) may offer some help. Oral β-carotene has been reported to help in erythrohepatic protoporphyria. Avoidance of drugs precipitating porphyria variegate is essential. In porphyria cutanea tarda, avoidance of alcohol is imperative, and venesection is helpful, as are small doses of chloroquine.

Referral to specialist is necessary to establish the diagnosis.

Long-term care. Patients will probably have to be seen at regular intervals, because of the associated complications which may occur with the various types of porphyria.

Xeroderma pigmentosa

Introduction

This is a rare hereditary disorder, the mode of inheritance being autosomal recessive. In xeroderma pigmentosa there is abnormal repair of DNA damaged by ultraviolet light due to enzyme deficiencies in the cells, which lead to subsequent malignant change in them.

Clinical features

Xeroderma pigmentosa usually presents at the age of 2–3 years and is characterized by erythema at the sites of exposure to ultraviolet light. There may be blister formation and the eyes are also photosensitive, giving rise to conjunctivitis and blepharitis. Irregular pigmentation, atrophic changes and telangiectasia soon appear. Keratoses and keratoacanthomata appear in early childhood, and usually before adolescence basal cell carcinomata, squamous cell carcinomata and melanomata may appear.

Problems

These are due to multiple skin tumours. Death usually occurs at a relatively early age owing to the skin malignancies which metastasize. The differential diagnosis includes porphyria and photosensitive eczema in the early stages.

Investigations and assessment

It is now possible to confirm the diagnosis by culture of skin fibroblasts after ultraviolet light irradiation, which show reduced ability to repair DNA. Prenatal diagnosis can be established in pregnant carriers by amniocentesis and is an indication for termination.

Management

Avoidance of sunlight by sunscreens and clothing is important. When keratoses begin to appear, topical 5-fluorouracil cream should be used. When malignant tumours appear they should be treated by surgery or curettage and cautery.

Referral to specialist is necessary for diagnosis and management.

Long-term care is necessary for early detection and treatment of malignant lesions.

IDIOPATHIC PHOTOSENSITIVE ERUPTIONS

Polymorphic light eruption

Introduction

This is the commonest photodermatosis.

Presentation

The disease is most commonly seen in women, and the commonest age of presentation is in late adolescence and young adulthood. The eruption usually occurs on all the exposed areas but surprisingly the face may be spared. The rash usually appears 2–48 hours after exposure to sunlight. The lesions may be small papules, erythema and occasionally blisters. The rash is itchy and tends to be excoriated. The problem may become less severe if the patients continue to be exposed to ultraviolet light and develop a suntan which protects the skin from further damage. The rash usually clears within a few days if no further exposure to sunlight occurs.

Problems

The eruption interferes with holidays and outdoor activities. The condition must be differentiated from other photosensitive disorders.

Assessment and investigation

No tests are diagnostic. Investigations may be necessary to exclude porphyria and systemic lupus erythematosus.

Management

Sunscreens may be helpful and should be tried. Avoidance of

sunlight as much as possible will minimize the problem but it limits the patient's social activities and holidays. Photochemotherapy (PUVA) will cause a deep tan and this offers protection during the summer months; maintenance treatment during the summer will be necessary to keep the tan.

The antimalarial drugs chloroquin and mepacrine are sometimes effective and may be taken for short periods such as a holiday. Long-term chloroquin is not advisable because of possible damage to the eye. Systemic steroids, prednisone 20mg daily, appear to be effective in preventing the eruption and are justified for a short period such as a holiday.

Long-term care may be necessary until the condition goes into spontaneous remission, which may not be until middle age.

Photosensitive eczema (actinic reticuloid)

Introduction

This is a condition seen mainly in middle-aged and elderly men. The name 'actinic reticuloid' was given to the condition because the histology resembled a reticulosis, but the condition is benign.

Clinical features

The eruption begins in the exposed areas, but after a time may spread to affect non-exposed areas and may even be generalized. The rash is red and scaly and there is thickening of the skin. Irritation is severe.

Problems

In the severe forms it appears that not only ultraviolet light but also visible light may aggravate the condition. Thus patients are unable to go out during the day, and have to draw the curtains during the day. Fluorescent lamps should be avoided.

The differential diagnosis includes contact eczema, photocontact eczema and, when widespread, endogenous eczema.

Assessment and investigation

Biopsy is often necessary to confirm the diagnosis. Patch tests and photo-patch tests are necessary to exclude exogenous factors.

Management

Light must be avoided as much as possible, and patients often have to do night work. Fluorescent lamps at home and at work have to be avoided. Sunscreens may offer some help. Potent topical steroids may clear the eruption, but weak ones are not usually effective. Systemic steroids are indicated if the condition becomes generalized or fails to respond to topical measures. Azathioprine has also been found to be effective, and can be used instead of, or in addition to, systemic steroids.

Referral to specialist is necessary for investigation and management.

Long-term care is necessary for supervision of treatment, as the condition is persistent.

Hutchinson's summer prurigo

Introduction

This is a relatively rare photodermatosis of unknown aetiology seen in children.

Clinical features

Characteristically the eruption begins as grouped papules on the lower half of the nose, cheeks and backs of the hands. Occasionally non-exposed areas are also affected. Although the eruption is most prominent in the summer it does not always clear in the winter. The problem may clear at puberty but this is not always so.

Problems

Other photodermatoses, particularly the porphyrias, have to be considered, but they usually present with erythema and blisters rather than papules.

Assessment and investigation

Tests to exclude porphyria and lupus erythematosus are necessary.

Management

Sunlight should be avoided and sunscreens should be used. Thalidomide has been reported to be effective in this particular dermatosis. Systemic steroids may be given for short periods, e.g. for a summer holiday.

Referral to specialist and long-term care are necessary for diagnosis and supervision of treatment.

PROTECTION OF THE SKIN FROM SUNLIGHT AND ARTIFICIAL LIGHT

Most, but not all, of the photodermatoses are due to ultraviolet light from the sun, and not to visible light. Ultraviolet light is divided into UVC (250–290nm), UVB (290–320nm) and UVA (320–400nm). UVC is completely absorbed in the earth's atmosphere, and UVB and UVA are partially absorbed. Thus the shorter the distance travelled through the atmosphere the less ultraviolet absorbed, i.e. at the equator. It should be remembered that some u.v. radiation will pass through cloud. Snow, sand and rippling water will also reflect u.v. radiation and thus increase the effect on the skin. Mountainous areas will have relatively more u.v. radiation, because the higher one goes, the less absorption of the u.v. light by the atmosphere. Thus photosensitive subjects should avoid visits to the tropics and mountains.

Patients who are sensitive to visible light (above 400 nm) should avoid all daylight apart from dusk and dawn. Patients are usually affected by the shorter wave blue–green part rather than the longer wave red–yellow part. Thus fluorescent lamps which give out the shorter wavelength visible light need to be avoided. Tungsten lamps should be used. Television sets and visual display units do not usually affect light-sensitive patients, but photocopying machines may be harmful.

Sunscreens

These may act by reflection or absorption of light. Absorbent sunscreens work by absorbing ultraviolet light and re-emitting it as insignificant quantities of heat. Absorbent sunscreens are *para*-aminobenzoic acid and its esters, cinnamates, salicylates and benzophenones. Absorbent sunscreens are mainly effective against UVB, and do not totally absorb UVA. Absorbent sunscreens are used in lotions and creams and some will persist despite washing, swimming or exercise. Reflectant sunscreens act by reflecting ultraviolet light and are therefore effective against UVA as well as UVB. They also reflect visible light. The two most commonly used reflectant sunscreens are titanium dioxide and zinc oxide. As both substances are white they are not cosmetically pleasing and they may have to be tinted. They tend to wash off in water.

Patients sensitive to UVB will be protected by absorbent sunscreens, those sensitive to UVA will only receive partial protection from absorbent ones, but reflectant sunscreens will protect against

UVB, UVA and visible light. Sunscreens are now readily available across the counter in pharmacies and cosmetics departments of large stores. They are now labelled with a sun protection factor (SPF) but this only refers to protection against UVB, which is the part of ultraviolet light which causes sunburn, and the SPF only refers to the absorbent sunscreens. The higher the SPF number, the greater the protection against UVB.

Natural protective mechanism

Sunlight not only causes increased pigmentation but also thickening of the epidermis. Both give protection against light. Thus patients who are able to work-through their photosensitivity often find they may be able to tolerate the sun once a tan develops.

PUVA (psoralens and UVA)

This will cause increased pigmentation and will afford protection against light. Patients who are very photosensitive will be unable to tolerate PUVA.

β-Carotene

This causes a yellow colour to the skin effective against UVA between 360–400nm and visible light. It is therefore effective for photodermatoses caused by visible light and UVA. These include polymorphic light eruption, erythrohepatic protoporphyria and solar urticaria.

Yellow plastic blinds

These are used to help screen-out shortwave visible light in patients sensitive to this part of the spectrum.

20

ICHTHYOSIS

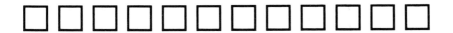

Ichthyosis comes from the Greek word *ichthys,* which means 'fish', as the skin in ichthyosis resembles fish scale. Ichthyosis is a disorder of keratinization. It may be hereditary or acquired. In hereditary ichthyosis the different genetic abnormalities lead to different biochemical processes and different clinical types of keratinization. Thus, hereditary ichthyosis forms a group of distinct clinical disorders with different clinical features and modes of inheritance.

ICHTHYOSIS VULGARIS

Introduction

This is the commonest type of ichthyosis and in its mildest forms it has been estimated that it affects one in 250 persons in the United Kingdom. The mode of inheritance is autosomal dominant. Ichthyosis vulgaris is not infrequently associated with atopy.

Clinical features

The disorder is not present at birth, and usually does not appear before the age of 3 months. It most commonly presents between the ages of 1 and 4 years. Ichthyosis is more common in cold, dry climates and may clear in warm, humid ones. Thus in the latter climate ichthyosis will not appear, but it will do so if the subject moves to a cold climate. In ichthyosis vulgaris the skin is dry and scaly, and has a 'cracked' appearance like crazy paving (Figure 36). The commonest sites of involvement are the limbs, with sparing of the flexures, and the back. In severe forms all the skin may be involved. In addition to the scaling there is often increased pigmentation. Keratosis pilaris on the back of the upper arms, and hyperkeratosis on the extensor surface of the knees and elbows may also be present.

Ichthyosis vulgaris often improves in adult life and may even clear.

Problems

Ichthyosis vulgaris is often associated with atopic eczema and thus patients present with features of both disorders complicating the clinical picture.

Patients with atopic eczema *per se* often have dry skin and this may have a similar appearance to mild ichthyosis. Other forms of hereditary ichthyosis can be differentiated by their different appearances. Acquired ichthyosis usually occurs in later life.

Assessment and investigation

The diagnosis is made on clinical grounds and biopsy is only rarely necessary.

Management

As cold tends to aggravate the condition it is important that the patient keep as warm as possible in winter with appropriate clothing. The face and hands should be protected from cold winds.

The patients should be told that when it comes to holidays warm weather will help and cold will make the condition worse.

Protection of the exposed skin from the elements with simple ointments such as emulsifying ointment B.P. may be helpful. The ointment tends to act as a simple barrier, the normal keratin barrier being deficient in ichthyosis.

The most helpful drug in ichthyosis vulgaris is 10% topical urea. This is applied in a simple cream base and a number of proprietary preparations (Calmurid and Aquadrate) are available. The cream should be applied every day after a bath. If the condition is not severe, less frequent application may suffice.

If atopic eczema is also present this should be treated with appropriate topical steroids prior to treatment with urea.

The retinoid, etretinate, has been used in ichthyosis vulgaris but the results have not been dramatic as in other forms of ichthyosis. Etretinate should be reserved for the more severely involved patients and those not improved with topical treatment.

Referral to hospital

This is usually only necessary for the diagnosis to be confirmed or established if there is any doubt. The more severely affected may have to be referred for management.

X-LINKED ICHTHYOSIS

Introduction

This disorder is only seen in males, and is inherited by a sex-linked recessive gene. It is associated with a deficiency in the skin of the enzyme steroid sulphatase, which is necessary for the metabolism of cholesterol for production of keratin in the skin.

It has been estimated that the incidence of X-linked ichthyosis is 1:6000.

Clinical features

X-linked ichthyosis may be present at birth or will appear in the first 3 months of life. The scales are large and brown and cover the whole of the body surface except for the palms and soles. It is more severe on the trunk, face, front of the neck and scalp. In adult life the disorder tends to be persistent and is most marked on the abdomen, lower legs and popliteal fossae. There is no associated follicular hyperkeratosis. Deep corneal opacities may occur.

Problems

X-linked ichthyosis has to be distinguished from the other hereditary forms of ichthyosis. The sparing of the palms and soles distinguishes it from lamellar ichthyosis and the flexural involvement distinguishes it from ichthyosis vulgaris.

X-linked ichthyosis tends to be persistent and may become worse in adult life. Treatment is palliative and not curative.

Assessment and investigation

The diagnosis is usually made on clinical grounds. Biopsy is confirmatory. Estimation of steroid sulphatase in the skin is not necessary for routine purposes.

Management

General measures

Like most forms of ichthyosis the condition tends to be worse in cold, dry climates, and thus protection of the skin with suitable clothing is helpful.

Topical preparations

Keratolytics (e.g. 2–5% salicylic acid) in an ointment base will reduce the scaling to a certain extent. 10% urea cream (Calmurid and Aquadrate) is helpful but is not as effective as in ichthyosis vulgaris. These preparations may be applied once or twice a day, particularly after bathing.

Recently it has been reported that as there is a deficiency of cholesterol in the skin, the topical application of cholesterol should be helpful, and 2% cholesterol in a base has indeed been shown to reduce the abnormal keratinization.

Systemic treatment

The retinoid, etretinate, has been used in X-linked ichthyosis but the results have not been encouraging.

Complications of treatment

Topical urea and cholesterol appear to be safe. Retinoids if used may cause a number of complications. These are described in the next section, on lamellar ichthyosis.

Referral to specialist

This is usually necessary for diagnosis and advice on treatment.

LAMELLAR ICHTHYOSIS

Introduction

This rare form of ichthyosis is transmitted by an autosomal recessive gene.

Clinical features

This disease is usually present at birth or will develop in the first 3 months of life. It begins as a generalized erythema and subsequently the skin becomes thickened and scaly. The scales tend to be large and there is involvement of the flexures, palms and soles. The flexural involvement may be the most severe; occasionally the disorder may present as a so-called 'collodion baby'. In this condition the baby is usually premature with shiny skin which feels hard and rigid. There is ectropion and a Cellophane-like membrane, and distortion of the face. Several days after birth the membrane sheds in large scales, and the underlying skin then gradually takes on the form of the ichthyosis; occasionally the child is stillborn.

In lamellar ichthyosis, ectropion is common and cortical cataracts may be present.

Problems

Lamellar ichthyosis must be distinguished from the other forms of ichthyosis. Lamellar ichthyosis tends to persist throughout life although there may be improvement in childhood.

Assessment and investigation

Biopsy may be necessary to establish the diagnosis. An ophthalmological opinion should be sought if the ectropion is severe and if there is doubt about cataracts.

Management

Topical

Keratolytics, such as 2–5% salicylic acid ointment, may decrease the degree of hyperkeratosis.

Systemic

The oral retinoid, etretinate, has been reported as being beneficial in this type of ichthyosis. The initial dose should be 0.5mg/kg body weight, and the dose should then be altered according to side-effects and clinical response.

Complications of treatment

Minor side-effects of retinoids include dry lips, nose bleeds and hair loss. Retinoids may cause liver damage and elevation of blood lipids, and these side-effects may limit their use. Retinoids are teratogenic and etretinate will persist in the body for up to 1 year after stopping of the drug. Thus pregnancy must be avoided during medication and for 1 year after stopping of the drug.

Referral to specialist

This is necessary for diagnosis and for supervision of treatment with the oral retinoids.

Long-term care

This will be necessary if patients choose to have treatment. Possible side-effects from systemic therapy will need to be assessed at regular intervals. Periodic eye assessment should also be carried out.

BULLOUS ICHTHYOSIFORM ERYTHRODERMA

Introduction

This is a rare form of ichthyosis transmitted by an autosomal dominant gene.

Clinical features

The skin is usually normal at birth but occasionally the presentation is that of a collodion baby. The onset is usually from birth up to 6 months. The infant develops attacks of redness, scaling and bullae. The bullae occur most frequently on the legs and become less frequent with age. The eruption may be generalized or become localized to the flexural regions. Other areas where localization may occur include the face, neck and back of the hands and feet. The skin in the affected areas is grossly thickened and hyperkeratotic, with deep ridging. The palms and soles may be involved. Bullous ichthyosiform erythroderma tends to improve with age and bulla formation becomes less. The condition may even clear around puberty.

Problems

Secondary infection of ruptured bullae may occur. The disorder has to be distinguished from other forms of ichthyosis, particularly the lamellar form. Other bullous disorders seen in childhood have also to be considered in the differential diagnosis and these include epidermolysis bullosa, bullous impetigo, and papular urticaria.

Assessment and investigation

Biopsy may be necessary to distinguish the condition from other forms of ichthyosis and bullous disorders.

Management

Topical

Simple keratolytics (2–5% salicylic acid ointment) will help to decrease the hyperkeratosis, but should not be applied to the bullous areas or where erosions have occurred. Lactic acid 5% in a cream base has also been used with beneficial results.

Systemic

Antibiotics are necessary if infection occurs once the bullae rupture. Retinoids, both isotretinoin and etretinate, have been used. These drugs help to clear the hyperkeratosis but do not suppress the bullae formation and may even aggravate them. It is too early to say which retinoid is the drug of choice.

Complications of treatment

These are mainly related to the retinoids and are as described in the previous section, on lamellar ichthyosis.

Referral to specialist

This will be necessary to establish the diagnosis and probably for supervision with treatment, if systemic treatment is chosen.

Long-term care

This will be necessary until the condition clears or ceases to trouble the patient.

ACQUIRED ICHTHYOSIS

Introduction

This is a type of ichthyosis which occurs due to underlying diseases, or patients taking nicotinic acid. The disorders which have been associated with acquired ichthyosis include Hodgkin disease, other lymphomas, carcinoma and mycosis fungoides. It has also been reported with malnutrition, liver damage and malabsorptive states. Ichthyosis also occurs in a small proportion of patients with lepromatous leprosy.

Clinical features

The scaling in acquired ichthyosis resembles that seen in ichthyosis vulgaris. The skin is dry and scaly with cracking but there is no thickening of the skin apart from the palms and soles.

Problems

Acquired ichthyosis has to be distinguished from dry, scaly skin seen in eczema where there may only be visible, minimal inflammatory changes. Ichthyosis vulgaris may be precipitated in somebody moving from a warm humid climate to a cold one.

Assessment and investigation

Examination may reveal signs of an underlying disease but if not, then patients should be investigated for evidence of the above disorders known to be associated with acquired ichthyosis.

Management

The underlying disorder should be treated, and the ichthyosis may well subside with symptomatic treatment of 10% urea cream.

Referral to specialist

This is necessary for investigation of the possible underlying condition.

21

DRUG ERUPTIONS

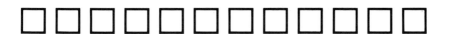

INTRODUCTION

It would be reasonable to state that any drug may cause a skin rash. The pattern and type of skin rash produced is variable although some drugs are more likely to produce certain types of eruption than others. The mechanism by which drugs produce skin lesions is not fully understood. It seems likely that there are two possible pathogenic pathways, first a direct 'toxic' effect on components of the skin, and second 'allergic' in which there is an antigen–antibody reaction. In the second type the drug itself may act as the antigen or it may combine with a hapten to form the antigen. Why some individuals develop skin rashes when taking drugs is not known, but host factors are obviously important and the development of rashes appears to be an idiosyncratic response on the part of the individual.

PRESENTATION

The appearance of the eruption is dependent on the primary site and nature of the pathological process in the skin. As a general rule a drug rash is suggested by the sudden onset of the eruption and is often widespread and symmetrical. There may be constitutional upset such as headache and fever. No medical history is complete without enquiring whether patients are taking drugs, and this includes self-medication with drugs which may be purchased at the chemist's shop without a prescription. The interval of time between taking the drug and the appearance of the rash may vary from a few hours to a few weeks. Although the skin lesions produced by reaction to drugs are extremely variable, certain patterns are more common and certain drugs are likely to give rise to certain types of eruption. These are described below.

Urticaria and angioneurotic oedema

The commonest drugs to cause urticarial eruptions are salicylates and penicillin. The eruption may occur within a few hours or be delayed for a few weeks after drug intake, particularly with penicillin. Occasionally there may be oedema of the tongue and laryngeal tissues, and in this instance the problem may prove fatal without immediate treatment.

Purpura

As happens with other causes of purpura, the eruption is most likely to appear first on the legs, but it may become generalized. The drugs most likely to produce purpura include thiazide diuretics, phenothiazines and isoniazid.

Maculopapular erythema

This is one of the more common types of drug rash. It is usually extensive and may become scaly, and progress to resemble exfoliative dermatitis. The antibiotics ampicillin and co-trimoxazole are the commonest cause of this type of rash.

Bullous eruptions

Non-specific bullous eruptions are seen with barbiturates, sulphonamides, iodides and bromides. The bullae tend to be large and tense and are more frequently found on the limbs than the trunk.

Toxic epidermal necrolysis

This is a relatively rare drug eruption. Originally the lesions begin as tender, red patches, which subsequently turn into flaccid blisters in which the whole of the roof of the blister sloughs off, leaving a red weeping area. The condition is usually self-limiting and clears within 2 weeks. If the condition is extensive, however, it may prove fatal. Toxic epidermal necrolysis has been induced by non-steroidal anti-inflammatory drugs, sulphonamides, barbiturates, phenytoin and dichloralphenazone (Welldorm).

Exfoliative dermatitis

This begins as red, scaly patches which gradually enlarge and increase in number to involve all the skin. The most common drug to cause this problem is gold. It has also been described with phenylbutazone, sulphonamides and sulphonylureas.

Lupus erythematosus

The typical skin lesions of systemic lupus erythematosus may be produced by penicillin, hydralazine, procainamide, griseofulvin, reserpine and phenylbutazone. Although the serological tests are positive for systemic lupus erythematosus, the disease is not severe when drug induced and has a good prognosis. There is rarely involvement of internal organs.

Acneiform eruption

This is a papular and pustular eruption usually on the face and upper trunk as found in acne. The drugs which tend to cause this problem are corticosteroids, androgens, oral contraceptives (mainly the progesterone-only preparations, or those low in oestrogen but with progesterones which have androgenic properties), iodides, fluorides, bromides and isoniazid.

Lichenoid eruptions

These often have features of both eczema and lichen planus and appear as violaceous scaly plaques most commonly on the trunk. The drugs most likely to cause this type of rash are the antimalarial drugs, chloroquin, mepacrine and quinine. In addition thiazide diuretics, heavy metals, phenothiazines and methyldopa may also induce this type of eruption.

Erythema multiforme

This eruption, including the severe form with involvement of the mucous membranes (Stevens–Johnson syndrome) may be caused by gold, phenylbutazone, phenytoin, sulphonylureas and sulphonamides.

Erythema nodosum

The eruption has been most commonly seen with sulphonamides and sulphonylureas.

Psoriasiform eruptions

Psoriasis has been precipitated or aggravated in susceptible individuals by lithium salts and chloroquin. Psoriasiform eruptions have also been caused by β-adrenergic blockers.

Photosensitivity

As the name implies, this type of rash occurs on the exposed areas
and is usually seen after exposure to strong sunlight. The eruption
may be mild with redness and scaling, or more severe with weeping
and crusting. Blister formation may also occur particularly with
nalidixic acid. Other drugs which cause photosensitivity include
the tetracyclines, particularly dimethylchlortetracycline, sulphonamides, thiazides and phenothiazines (particularly chlorpromazine).

Porphyria cutanea tarda may be precipitated by certain drugs,
including oestrogens and griseofulvin.

Fixed drug eruptions

In this disorder the skin lesions are produced at the same sites
every time the drug is taken. Fixed drug eruptions usually occur
with drugs which are taken intermittently. The lesion usually
begins as a red patch, and this is often followed by blister formation, crusting and weeping. As the lesions heal there is often
residual pigmentation. Fixed drug eruption is most commonly seen
with phenolphthalein (found in laxatives), sulphonamides, barbiturates, quinine, tetracyclines and phenylbutazone.

PROBLEMS

Drug eruptions have to be distinguished from the rash that they are
often mimicking. The diagnosis is suggested by a short history,
often the rash being extensive and symmetrical, and a history of
recent drug intake. In patients who develop drug eruptions, the
rash usually appears in the patient soon after starting the drug
rather than in a patient who has been taking it continuously for any
length of time.

ASSESSMENT AND INVESTIGATION

Unfortunately there are no worthwhile tests for proving that a rash is caused by a particular drug. In severely affected patients and those with constitutional upset, it is wise to have a full blood count, liver function tests and urine analysis, to see if other organs are also involved.

MANAGEMENT

If a drug rash is suspected it is important that the offending drug is stopped as soon as possible. If a patient is taking several drugs it may not be possible to determine which drug is the most likely one to have caused the eruption but, as can be seen from the above, certain drugs are more likely to cause rashes than others, and thus these should be stopped first. If the drugs have been stopped but it is subsequently necessary to continue them, then if possible one drug at a time should be reintroduced, the drugs least likely to have caused the rash being given first. If it is obvious which drug caused the rash, but therapy needs to be continued, then a drug which has a similar action but different structure should be chosen if possible. One of the commonest group of drugs to cause rashes is the antibiotics, and it is usually possible to find one which can be substituted for the offender. As a general rule, if a particular antibiotic – e.g. pencillin – has caused the eruption, it is advisable not to use one from the same group.

Usually if a drug has caused an eruption it may have the same effect in the future, but this is not always the case. In some instances it appears that the condition being treated may determine if a rash appears, e.g. ampicillin always causes a rash in glandular fever, but it may be taken once the disease is no longer active.

If a particular drug, out of a group which the patient is taking, is considered essential for treatment, but it is not known if it is the particular offending one, the only way of proving whether it caused the rash is by challenge. A small single dose is given and a sufficient period of time (may be up to 2 weeks) should be allowed to see if a rash appears.

Whether any treatment is given for the actual rash will depend on its severity. If the eruption is mild then no treatment is necessary. Most drug eruptions are self-limiting and clear within 2 weeks. If the eruption is predominantly urticarial, oral antihistamines should be given. Irritation is often a symptom with drug eruptions and, if it is severe, oral antihistamines are indicated. If there is epidermal involvement as manifested by scaling or crusting, topical steroid creams or lotions may decrease the inflammation and irritation. If the eruption is severe with blisters and erosions, as may be seen in the Stevens–Johnson syndrome or toxic epidermal necrolysis, a systemic steroid should be given. Intravenous therapy may be necessary in extensive involvement of toxic epidermal necrolysis to maintain electrolyte balance.

It is important that patients should be told which drug is responsible for the rash and if possible they should carry this information with them in case of emergencies. Their notes should be clearly marked with an indication of the particular drug sensitivity.

Referral to specialist

This is only necessary if there is doubt about diagnosis or the problem is severe enough to warrant admission to hospital.

22

PRURITUS

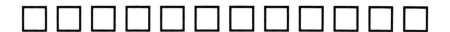

INTRODUCTION

Pruritus, or itch, is a subjective symptom that occurs in many skin conditions, especially those involving sensitivity reactions and histamine release, most typically atopic eczema, urticaria, infestations, candidal infection and insect bites.

Pruritus may also occur in association with systemic conditions such as the uraemia of chronic renal failure, obstructive liver diseases, particularly biliary cirrhosis, thyroid disease, diabetes, Hodgkin disease, chronic lymphatic leukaemia, some carcinomata, and polycythaemia.

Other situations that may contribute to pruritus are psychogenic disturbance, dry skin associated with old age, excessive sweating and chafing, climatic change, pregnancy and the contraceptive pill, some of these probably being superimposed on some degree of atopy.

MANAGEMENT

In the absence of any obvious associated skin disease a careful search for scabies burrows and papules should be made. Pediculosis may also cause pruritus but is less common. Intestinal parasitic infestations, such as hookworm or roundworm, onchocerciasis and filariasis may also present with pruritus.

In obstructive biliary disease it is thought that pruritus is caused by excess deposition of bile salts in the skin. Pruritus may be the presenting feature of biliary cirrhosis and precede other symptoms of the disease by 1–2 years. Similarly in Hodgkin disease, pruritus may precede other symptoms and signs by as much as 2 years.

In diabetes a generalized pruritus has been reported but usually the symptom is localized and secondary to candidal infection, most typically as pruritus vulvae.

If the underlying cause of a pruritus is not clear, then the following investigations may be helpful: full blood count and ESR; liver, renal and thyroid function blood tests; CXR; urine and stool analysis; mitochondrial antibodies for possible biliary cirrhosis.

Treatment is management of the underlying condition. Systemic antihistamines may be useful whatever the cause of pruritus. Topical applications containing steroids should only be used when clearly appropriate, and not indiscriminately.

In biliary cirrhosis administration of the resin cholestyramine may ease pruritus by reducing the level of bile salts deposited in the skin.

In prurigo nodularis, a skin condition of unknown cause characterized by itchy, hard, scaly nodules in areas accessible to excoriation, it has been found that a few patients have an associated gluten-sensitive enteropathy, and treatment with a gluten free diet in these cases improves the dermatosis and reduces pruritus.

23

CUTANEOUS MANIFESTATIONS OF METABOLIC DISEASE

□ □ □ □ □ □ □ □ □ □ □ □

DIABETES MELLITUS

The commonest skin problem associated with this disease is infection, usually due to either staphylococci or *Candida albicans* and such infection may be a presenting sign of the diabetes. Vascular disease secondary to diabetes can cause ischaemic skin changes sometimes leading to ulcers and gangrene, and diabetic neuropathy may lead to neurotrophic ulcers.

Necrobiosis lipoidica is an eruption which begins as brownish-coloured papules and plaques, that may occur on the shins both in overt and latent diabetics. The lesions become atrophic and may ulcerate. The condition is thought to be related to small vessel disease.

Granuloma annulare has been traditionally associated with diabetes although it is realized now that patients with this skin condition have no higher incidence of diabetes than does the general population. Lesions start as firm papules or nodules in the dermis, usually on the backs of hands and fingers (Figure 37), on extensor surfaces of the elbows and knees or around the ankles, the lesions extending in annular pattern with central healing, and appearing indurated, granulomatous and non-scaling. The eruption usually clears spontaneously in 2 years, but it can be treated if necessary by intralesional injection of triamcinolone.

Other skin lesions common in diabetics are lipoatrophy at the site of insulin injections (less usual with the modern purer insulins) and xanthomatosis.

Xanthomata

These are localized deposits of lipids that may occur in diabetes mellitus, hypothyroidism, nephrotic syndrome, liver disease (usually biliary cirrhosis), and the six types of primary hyperlipidaemia, different forms of lesion occurring in each type.

Xanthelasma is the commonest form of xanthoma and presents as a yellowish-white plaque on the upper eyelid or just below the lower eyelid, usually medially. The lesion can occur in Type IIA primary hyperlipidaemia, many of the secondary hyperlipidaemias, and also in subjects who have no generalized biochemical disorder.

Nodular xanthomata usually occur on extensor surfaces of limbs, particularly over the joints, and may be as large as 2cm in diameter. Papular xanthomata usually occur on the trunk or buttocks and occasionally appear rapidly over a few weeks as a crop of numerous small papules – when they are known as 'eruptive xanthomata'. Plaque xanthomata occur at many sites but most commonly along the tendon sheaths.

Treatment of xanthomata and reduction of hyperlipidaemia is allied to the overall management of the specific underlying disorder. In patients with xanthelasmata in whom no biochemical disorders are found the lesions can be removed by surgery, or electrocautery under local anaesthetic.

GOUT

Gouty tophi are deposits of urate which present as nodules on the ears, hands, or extensor surfaces of limb joints. The overlying skin is fixed to the nodule and occasionally breaks, leading to ulceration and discharge. Tophi are rare in the absence of arthritis and usually indicate chronic gout with renal involvement. The location of tophi and the asymmetry of the arthritis distinguish the lesions from rheumatoid nodules and Heberden's nodes. The hyperuricaemia of gout is often associated with hyperlipidaemia and xanthomatosis.

24

ERYTHEMA NODOSUM

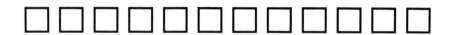

INTRODUCTION

Erythema nodosum is a cutaneous hypersensitivity reaction, essentially a vasculitis, manifest as red tender nodules or plaques usually occurring on the shins, but occasionally on the backs of the legs and on the extensor surfaces of the arms, and rarely on the neck. The most common precipitating causes of the condition are streptococcal infection, primary tuberculosis, sarcoidosis, and drugs, most often sulphonamides. Less frequent causes of erythema nodosum include fungal infections, meningococcal septicaemia, Crohn's disease, ulcerative colitis, and lymphogranuloma venereum. In some patients no cause is found.

CLINICAL FEATURES

The lesions vary in size from 1 to 10cm in diameter, and occasionally become confluent. Initially the nodules or plaques are painful, red, and tender, but after 2–3 weeks they become less painful, turn purple, and involute. Lesions do not necessarily appear simultaneously and tend to arise in crops, but all lesions should have cleared within a month of onset.

MANAGEMENT

The most important part of management is diagnosis and treatment of the underlying condition (if appropriate). After careful history and examination the most useful investigations are CXR, blood count and ESR, anti-streptolysin titre, throat swab, and skin tests for tubercle and sarcoid. Treatment of the eruption itself usually consists of rest and mild analgesics, but sometimes the illness is more severe and requires bedrest, stronger analgesics, and occasionally systemic corticosteroids. Investigations to determine the precipitating cause of the condition must be started at an early stage and certainly should be completed before treatment with steroids is contemplated.

25

CUTANEOUS VASCULITIS

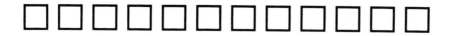

Cutaneous vasculitis is a broad term implying inflammatory damage to arterioles and small arteries in the skin. The condition usually presents as multiple purpuric papules and/or blisters if superficial vessels are involved, or as deeper firm nodules or plaques if larger deeper vessels are involved (e.g. erythema nodosum). The condition may be associated with a chronic reticular cyanosis known as 'livedo reticularis'. As with other causes of purpura the commonest site for cutaneous vasculitis is the lower legs.

Most cases of cutaneous vasculitis are of unknown cause although damage by immune complexes appears to be a key factor in many instances, as it is in those cases of vasculitis which are known to be secondary to such conditions as infection, drug toxicity and connective tissue disease (e.g. polyarteritis nodosa).

Treatment of the vasculitis if it is severe or chronic, consists of systemic corticosteroids, and possibly immunosuppressive therapy or plasma exchange.

Conditions exhibiting cutaneous vasculitis may be listed as follows.

(1) *Cutaneous only:*
  (a) Chilblains
  (b) Idiopathic cutaneous vasculitis
  (c) Allergic vasculitis (drugs, foods)
  (d) Cutaneous polyarteritis
  (e) Erythema induratum (Bazin's disease)
  (f) Erythema nodosum
  (g) Idiopathic capillaritis
  (h) Nodular vasculitis
  (i) Panniculitis
  (j) Pityriasis lichenoides

(2) *Cutaneous/systemic:*
  (a) Idiopathic cutaneous/systemic vasculitis
  (b) Henoch–Schönlein purpura
  (c) Polyarteritis nodosa
  (d) Rheumatoid arthritis
  (e) Systemic lupus erythematosus (SLE)
  (f) Wegner's granulomatosis
  (g) Waldenström's hypergammaglobulinaemic purpura

26

PURPURA

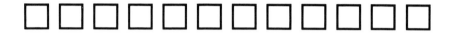

Purpura is discoloration of the skin or mucous membrane due to extravasated blood cells, as distinct from erythema which is due to capillary dilatation; pressure with a glass slide will blanch erythema but have no effect on purpura.

Purpuric lesions tend to be more purple than red, but later they become a reddish-brown colour. They vary in size from a few millimetres (petechiae) to several centimetres (ecchymoses or bruises). When secondary to a vasculitis, purpura may be raised, bullous, or ulcerated. Lesions are most common on the legs due to relatively high venous back pressure and capillary stasis.

Purpura is caused by either (1) a disorder of the blood or (2) a disorder of the blood vessel wall. Occasionally a condition causes disorder both in blood and vessel wall. Although the underlying disease is often identifiable some cases turn out to be idiopathic.

If the diagnosis of the condition causing purpura is not clinically obvious the following investigations may be helpful: FBC, differential WBC, platelet count, clotting studies, plasma protein electrophoresis, cryoglobulins, RA latex, ANF and DNA binding.

Most of the conditions causing purpura are subjects for haematology or general medicine texts. Table 26.1 provides a broad classification.

Table 26.1

Disorders of blood	Disorders of blood vessels
Thrombocytopenia:	Heredity
Idiopathic	Old age (senile purpura)
Drugs	Steroids
Leukaemia and carcinoma	Trauma/obstruction
Systemic lupus	Scurvy
erythematosus	Vasculitis (Allergic papular purpura)
Hypersplenism	Henoch–Schönlein purpura
Uraemia	Eczema
Other blood disorders:	Stasis/cold injury
Disseminated	Embolic phenomena (e.g. subacute
intravascular	bacterial endocarditis
coagulation	Idiopathic capillaritis
Drugs	
Dysprotinaemia	
Cryoglobulinaemia	
Infections	

27
LUPUS ERYTHEMATOSUS, SCLERODERMA, DERMATOMYOSITIS

☐ ☐ ☐ ☐ ☐ ☐ ☐ ☐ ☐ ☐ ☐ ☐

CHRONIC DISCOID LUPUS ERYTHEMATOSUS

This disorder affects men and women equally and usually commences in early or middle adult life. The commonest site is the face, but lesions may occur on scalp, ears, neck and hands and occasionally on arms and upper trunk. The eruption is usually asymmetrical and tends to appear for the first time after exposure to sunlight.

The lesion starts as a well-defined, slightly scaly, red plaque, with follicular dilation and 'plugging' by scales of keratin. The plaque may vary in size from 0.5 to 3 cm, and may merge with other plaques to involve the entire forehead or cheek. As the condition progresses the skin becomes atrophic and scarring occurs (Figure 38). Ulceration may occur as a late complication and, if it is chronic, squamous cell carcinoma may develop. On the lips and the vagina, erosions occur. On the scalp there is associated hair loss due to destruction of hair follicles. Eventually the condition becomes 'burnt out', and manifests as white patches of thickened scar tissue.

Treatment includes avoidance of sunlight, powerful topical steroids, occasionally systemic steroids if lesions are resistant, and antimalarial drugs such as chloroquine, although this is used rarely now because of possible corneal and retinal side-effects.

179

SYSTEMIC LUPUS ERYTHEMATOSUS (SLE)

This is a systemic disorder which may have skin manifestations, but is otherwise characterized by fatigue, fever, arthropathy, nephritis and pleural and pericardial effusions. The classical erythematous 'butterfly' rash over the nose and malar prominences occurs in about 50% of cases, and may extend to all the exposed areas, and occasionally become generalized, involving unexposed areas. Unlike those of chronic discoid lupus erythematosus, lesions do not become atrophic and scarred, and the main residual sign is hyperpigmentation.

Other cutaneous signs of the disease are possible hair loss, telangiectasia on the posterior nail folds, and splinter haemorrhages on the nail bed. Knees and elbows may show erythema, telangiectasia and scaling. Also, there might be purpura due to thrombocytopenia.

Serological studies show the presence of antinuclear antibodies and immunofluorescent study of skin biopsies shows deposition of immunoglobulins in the region of the basement membrane.

Treatment of systemic lupus erythematosus varies with the extent of the disease, systemic steroids tending to be used more for the acute stages, and the immunosuppressive drug azathioprine for the chronic phases. The disease runs a variable course but is usually chronic with intermittent exacerbations, with renal involvement as the most likely cause of death.

SCLERODERMA

As with lupus erythematosus there is a localized cutaneous form, called morphoea, and a systemic form.

Morphoea consists of a hardened plaque in the dermis with overlying atrophic epidermis, seen as a white patch with surrounding violaceous hue which later becomes pigmented. If the face is affected there may be underlying atrophy of the muscles. Lesions tend to gradually resolve over a 5–10-year period.

Systemic scleroderma may cause disturbances in all systems due to a generalized alteration in collagen. Raynaud's phenomenon may precede the more obvious signs of the condition by a number of years, but eventually the skin becomes tightened and shiny in appearance and the former may lead to deformity of the face and fingers. Cutaneous calcinosis is common in the fingertips causing hard nodules or ulcers. Macular telangiectasia on the face are common.

The course of the disease is variable, life expectancy varying from a few months to over 30 years, but 50% of sufferers die within 5 years, usually from renal failure, cardiac dysrhythmias or intestinal perforation. Hypertension and proteinuria secondary to renal involvement are bad prognostic signs, and steroids tend to make the hypertension worse; indeed, no drug has been shown to improve the condition significantly. Simple measures such as avoidance of cold, stopping smoking, and physiotherapy for arms and hands are the mainstay of treatment.

DERMATOMYOSITIS

This is a collagen disorder involving the skin and skeletal muscle. It may present in childhood or adult life, and in adults the condition is associated with internal malignancy in about 50% of cases.

Skin lesions usually begin as purplish, sometimes oedematous, erythema around the eyes. The rash may become generalized, scaly or blistering, and eventually patchy and atrophic. Calcinosis tends to occur around the joints (usually knees and elbows) and is commoner in childhood cases.

Muscles are affected around the shoulders, upper arms, pelvic girdle and thighs, at first causing weakness and later gross wasting. The diagnosis is usually confirmed by muscle enzyme and electromyogram studies.

The course of the disease is extremely variable, occasionally causing only a transient illness but more often becoming a chronic disease with exacerbations, eventually either burning itself out or leading to death from respiratory failure or from associated malignancy.

Systemic corticosteroids and cytotoxics provide the main therapies. If there is an associated carcinoma which is operable, resection of the tumour may lead to a remission of the dermatomyositis.

28

HYPERHIDROSIS

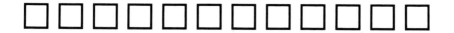

INTRODUCTION

Essential hyperhidrosis is excessive sweating when no obvious cause can be found.

CLINICAL FEATURES

This type of hyperhidrosis usually affects the emotional sweat areas, i.e. the axillae, palms and soles. Usually only one of these sites is involved.

The condition may begin in childhood, adolescence or early adult life. Essential hyperhidrosis tends to last a number of years but to disappear around middle age. In its severe forms it may lead to severe embarrassment and difficulty at work. When the axillae are involved the clothes are stained and the condition may literally rot certain materials. When the hands are involved any work handling paper becomes difficult and patients may have to look for alternative employment. When the soles are affected socks and shoes may be rotted away.

PROBLEMS

It is important to exclude other causes of excessive sweating, particularly hyperthyroidism, anxiety state and chronic infections such as brucellosis, tuberculosis and malaria. Rarer causes include phaeochromocytoma and disorders affecting the hypothalamus.

INVESTIGATIONS

If there is any doubt about the diagnosis, investigations to exclude other causes of hyperhidrosis will have to be carried out.

MANAGEMENT

The simplest and most effective treatment for essential hyperhidrosis is aluminium chloride solution. A high concentration is necessary, usually 25% of an alcoholic solution of aluminium chloride hexahydrate. A proprietary preparation containing 20% aluminium chloride (Driclor) is now available. The frequency of application varies between individuals and more frequent application is usually necessary on the palms and soles. Initially patients should be advised to apply the lotion on alternate nights and let it dry before going to bed. Contact with clothing should be avoided until the lotion has dried. Once sweating has been controlled the frequency of application should be decreased; a number of patients find weekly application sufficient to inhibit sweating. Aluminium chloride is an irritant and may cause mild eczema in the axillae if frequent application is necessary. This reaction can usually be controlled by 1% hydrocortisone cream. If sweating from the palms and soles cannot be controlled by the application of aluminium chloride, then soaking in the solution for 10–15 minutes should be tried and this may well be effective.

Since aluminium chloride has come into use for hyperhidrosis, surgical treatments are very rarely necessary. Excision of the axillary skin for axillary hyperhidrosis is an effective treatment and if carried out correctly has a low incidence of sequelae. Sympathectomy is probably not justified because of the side-effects that would have to be endured.

29

TOPICAL STEROIDS

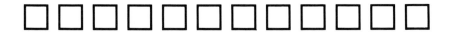

These are the drugs most widely used in dermatology and if employed correctly they are highly effective and safe. It is most important to appreciate that there is a considerable range of potency between the weakest and strongest topical steroid currently available, and the doctor prescribing the steroid should be aware of the potency of the drug (Table 29.1). Topical steroids are now arbitrarily divided into four groups: group I – weak; group II – moderate; group III – strong; and group IV – very strong. It is sufficient for the practising physician to learn one proprietary preparation from each group.

Side-effects from topical steroids are usually of a local nature and are due to their causing atrophy of the collagen and inhibiting fibroblasts and thus the formation of new collagen. Clinically this is manifest as thinning of the skin, telangiectasia (Figure 39), striae (Figure 40), and spontaneous bruising and purpura. Systemic side-effects are suppression of the pituitary adrenal axis and very rarely retention of fluid and Cushingoid features. Systemic side-effects are only seen with the use of large quantities of very strong fluid topical steroids.

Local side-effects are directly proportional to duration of use and strength of the steroid. Important factors influencing side-effects, however, are the thickness of the skin (it is different in different parts of the body) and moisture of the skin (increased moisture is found in intertriginous areas). Thus, as a general rule, strong and very strong steroids should not be used on the face (thin skin) and in the axillae, groins, perianal skin and submammary regions (intertriginous areas).

Table 29.1   Examples of topical steroid preparations of varying strengths

Strength	Generic name	Proprietary name
Group IV		
Very strong	Clobetasol propionate	Dermovate
Group III		
Strong	Betamethasone	Betnovate
	Beclomethasone dipropionate	Propaderm
	Diflucortolone valerate	Nerisone
	Fluclorolone acetonide	Topilar
	Fluocinolone acetonide	Synalar
	Fluocinonide	Metosyn
	Halcinonide	Halciderm
Group II		
Moderate	Clobetasone butyrate	Eumovate
	Flurandrenolone	Haelan
Group 1		
Weak	Hydrocortisone	Efcortelan
		Hydrocortistab
		Hydrocortisyl

Index

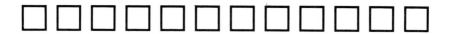

189